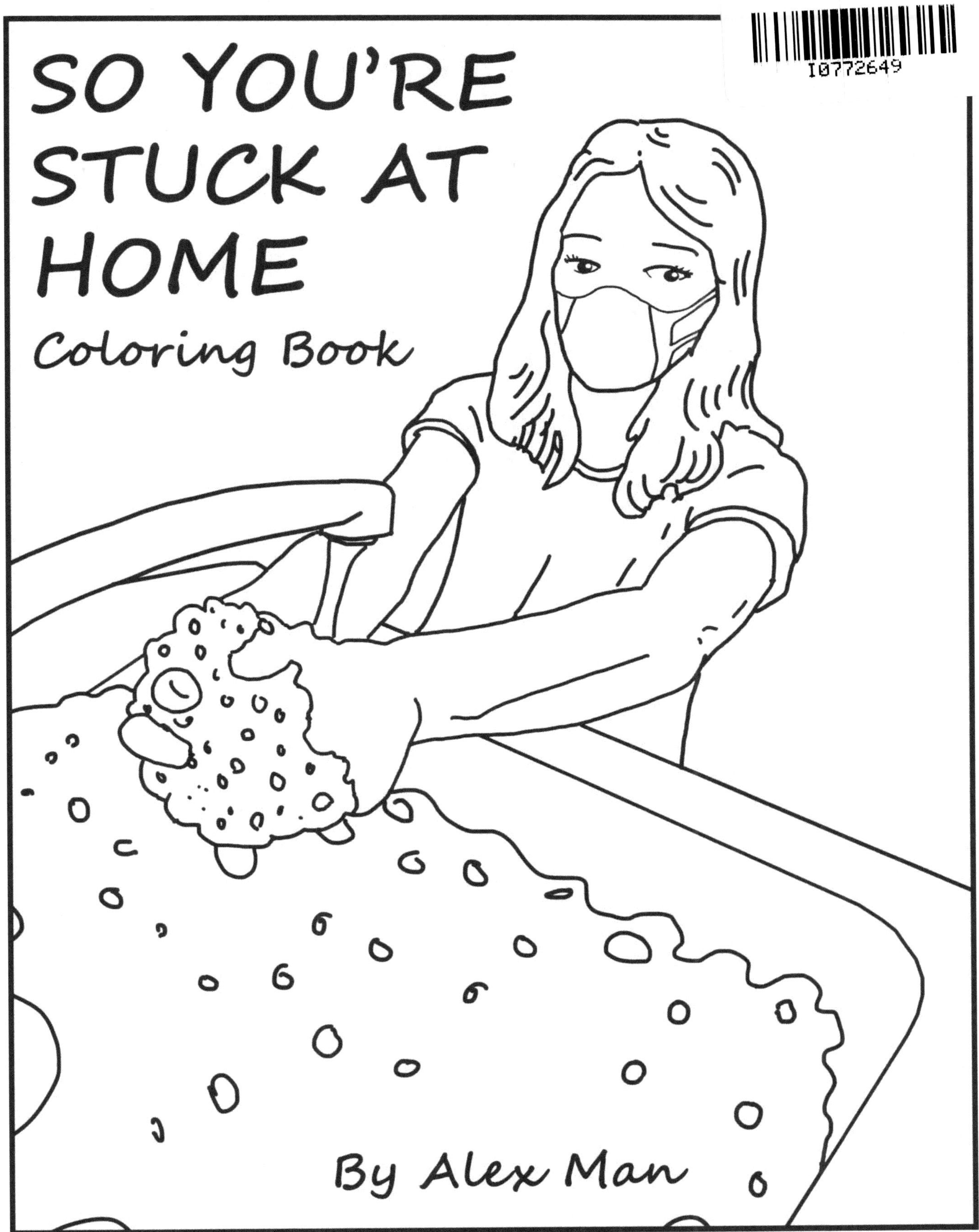

SO YOU'RE STUCK AT HOME
Coloring Book
By Alex Man
I0772649

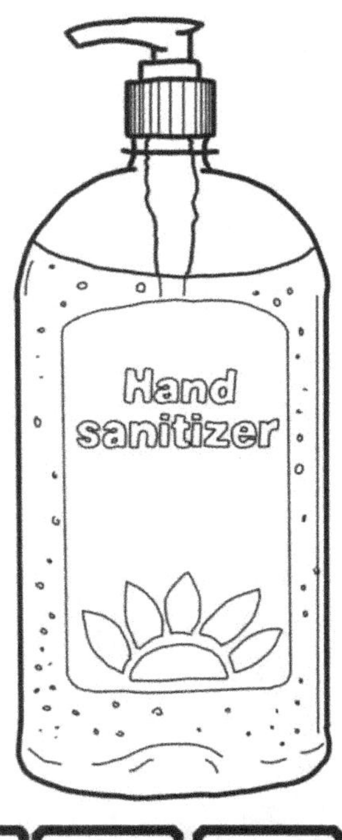


KEEP
CALM
AND
CLEAN YOUR
HANDS

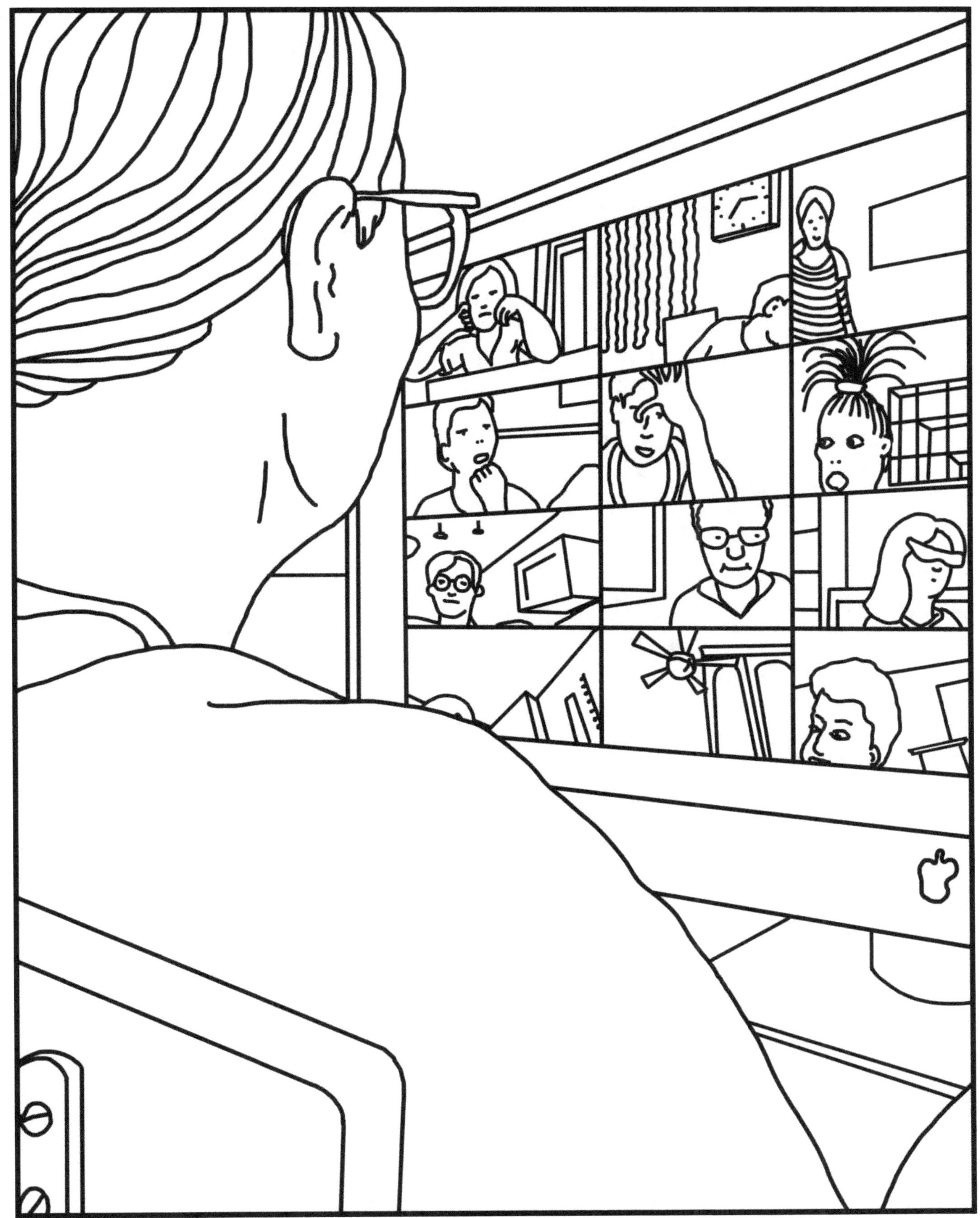

# Cough or sneeze? Elbow please

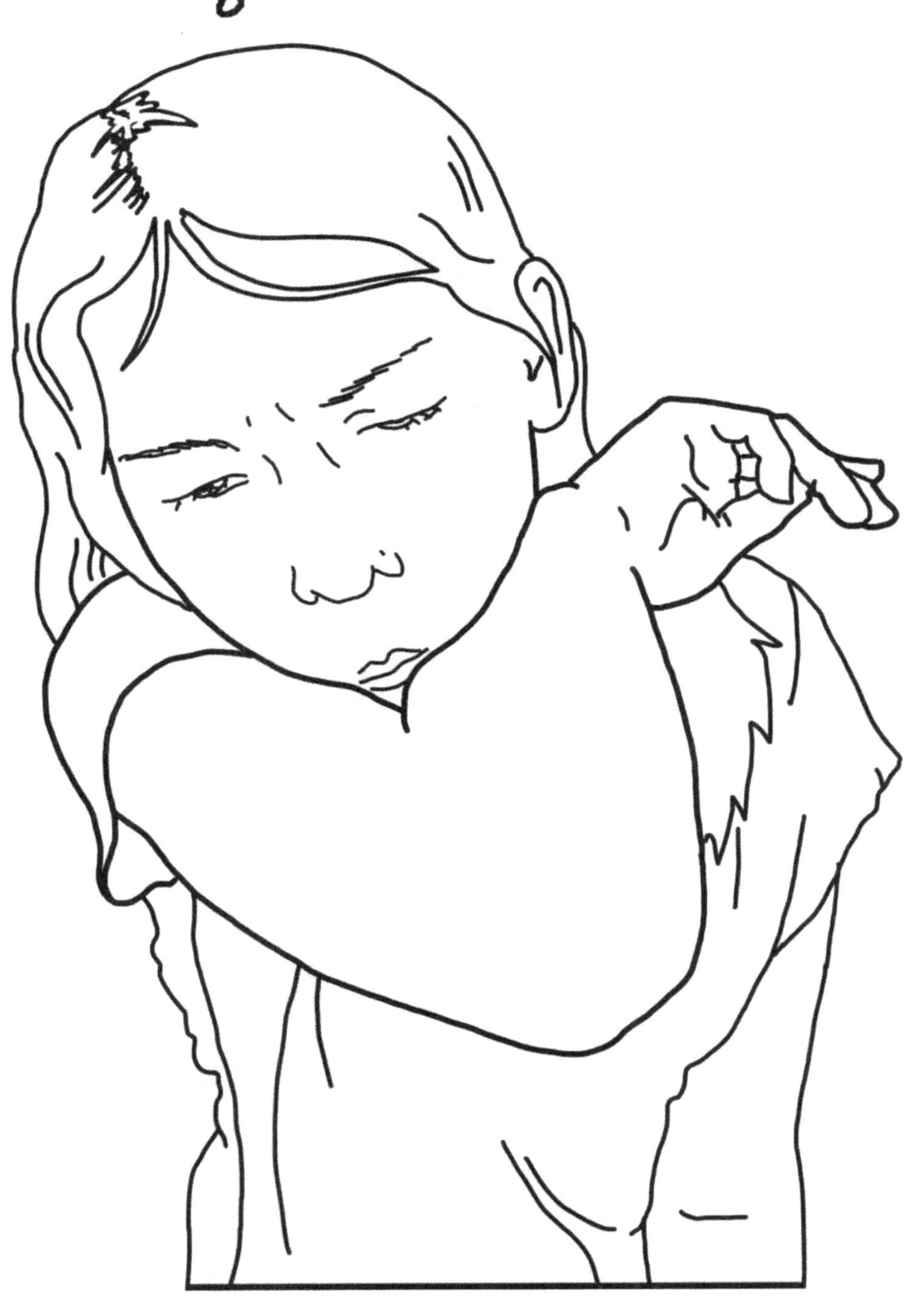

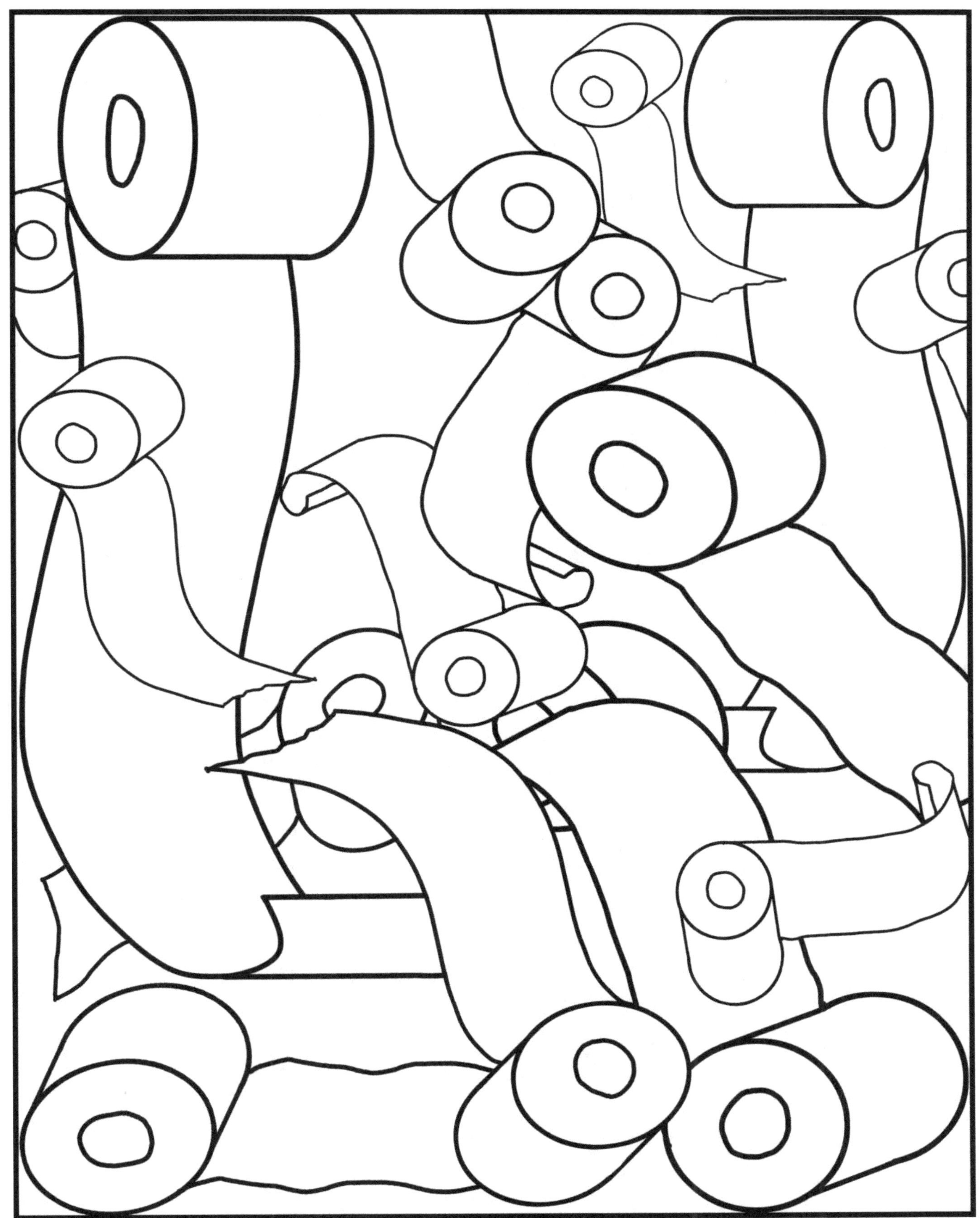

Feel Better!
tissue

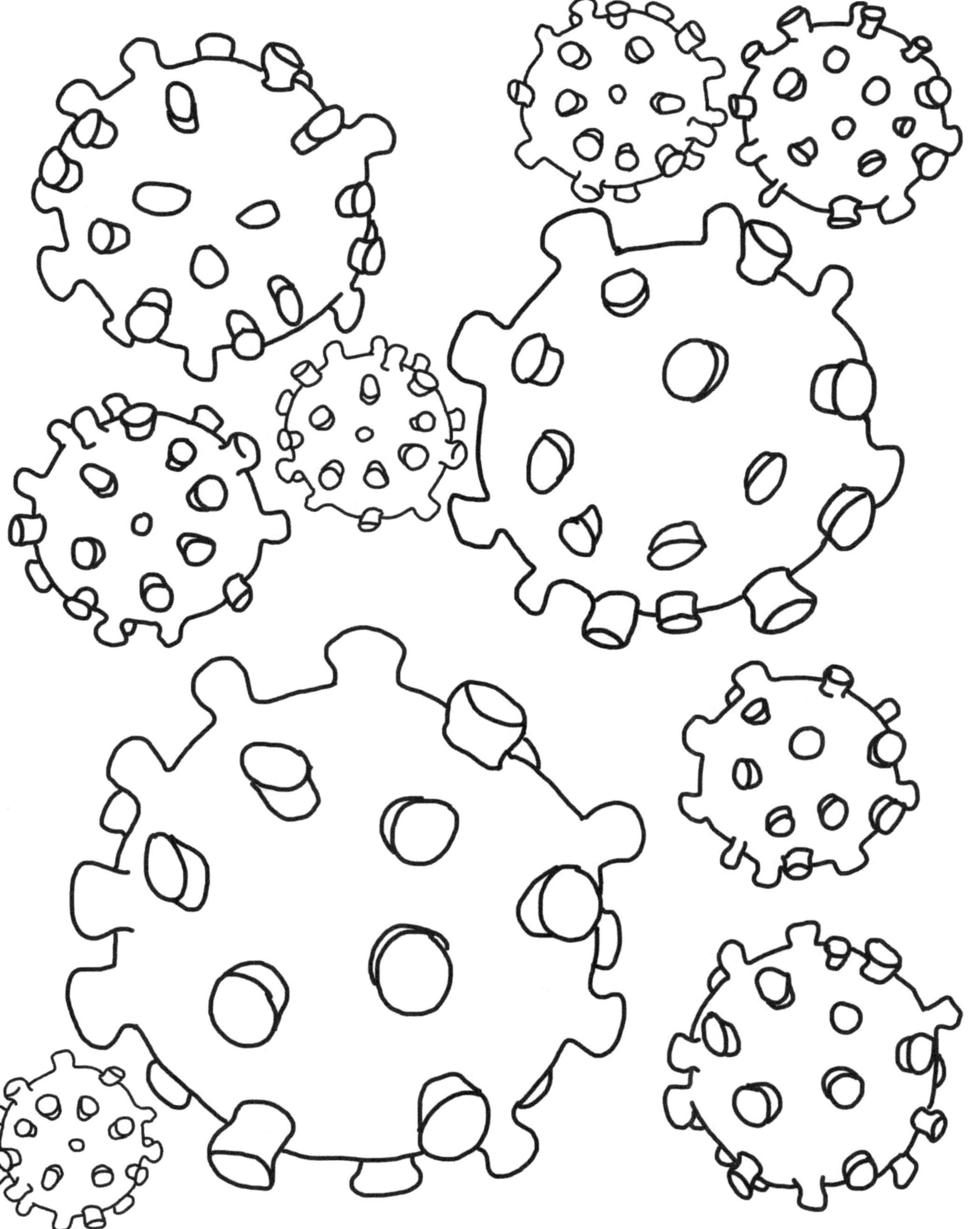

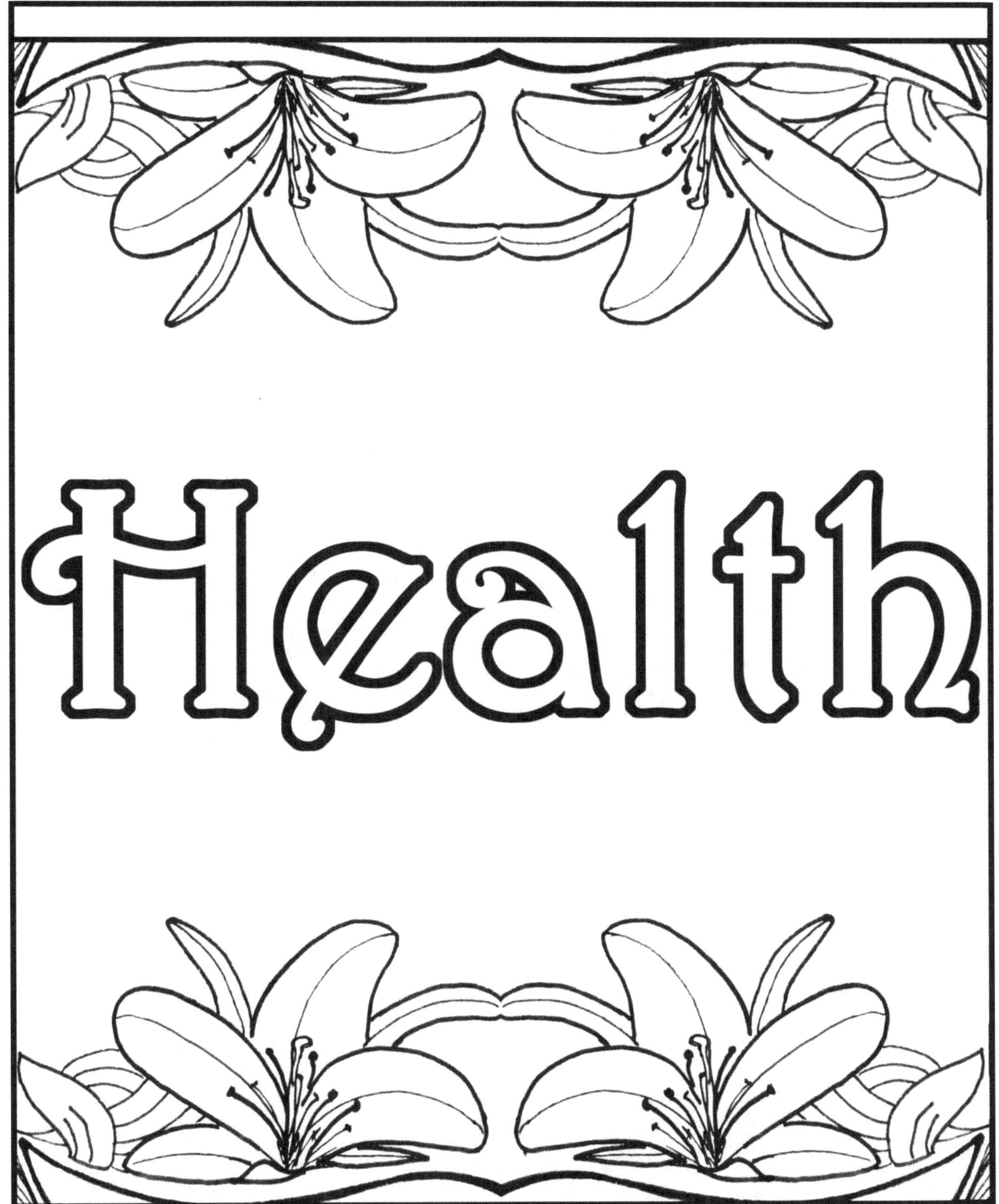
Health

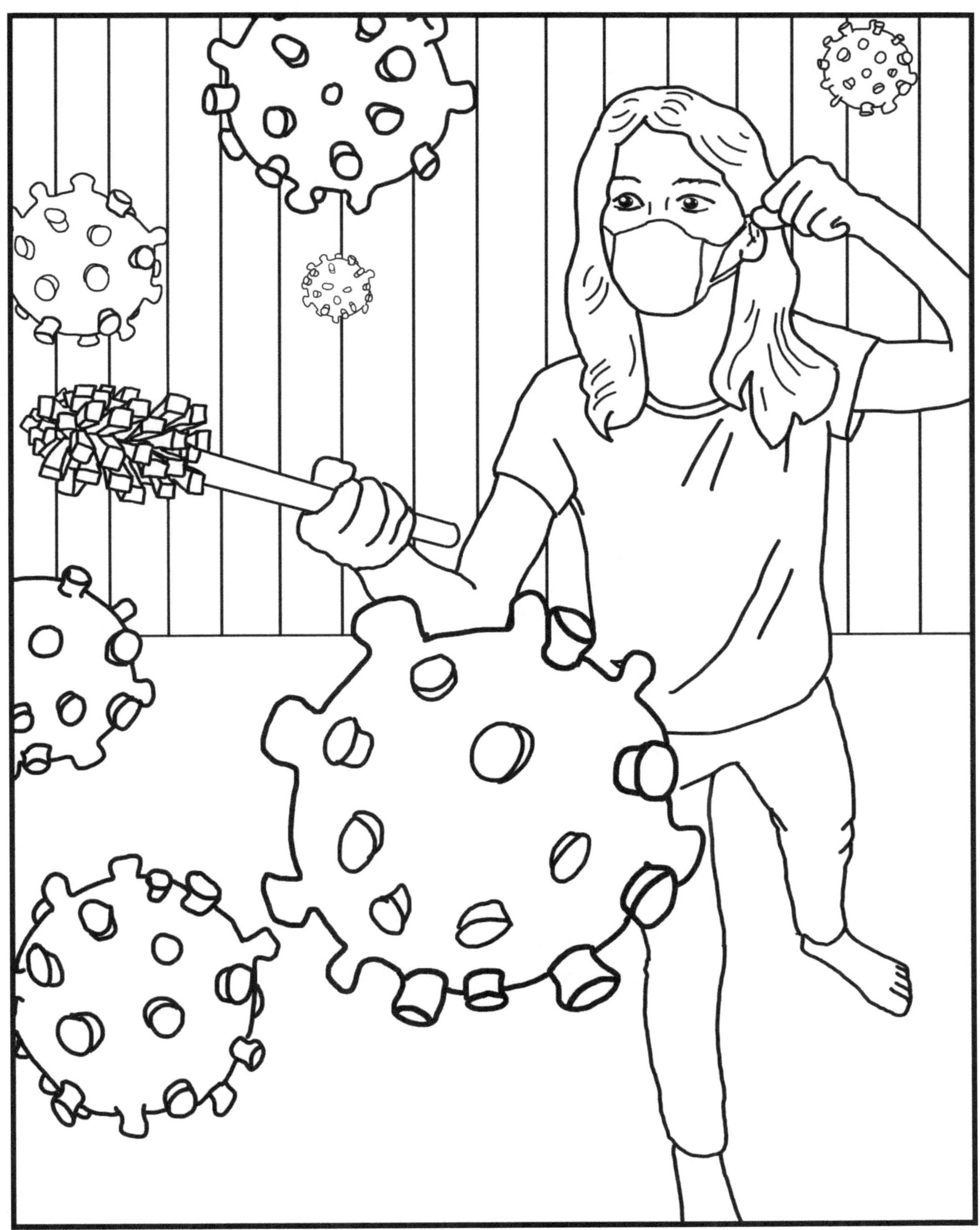

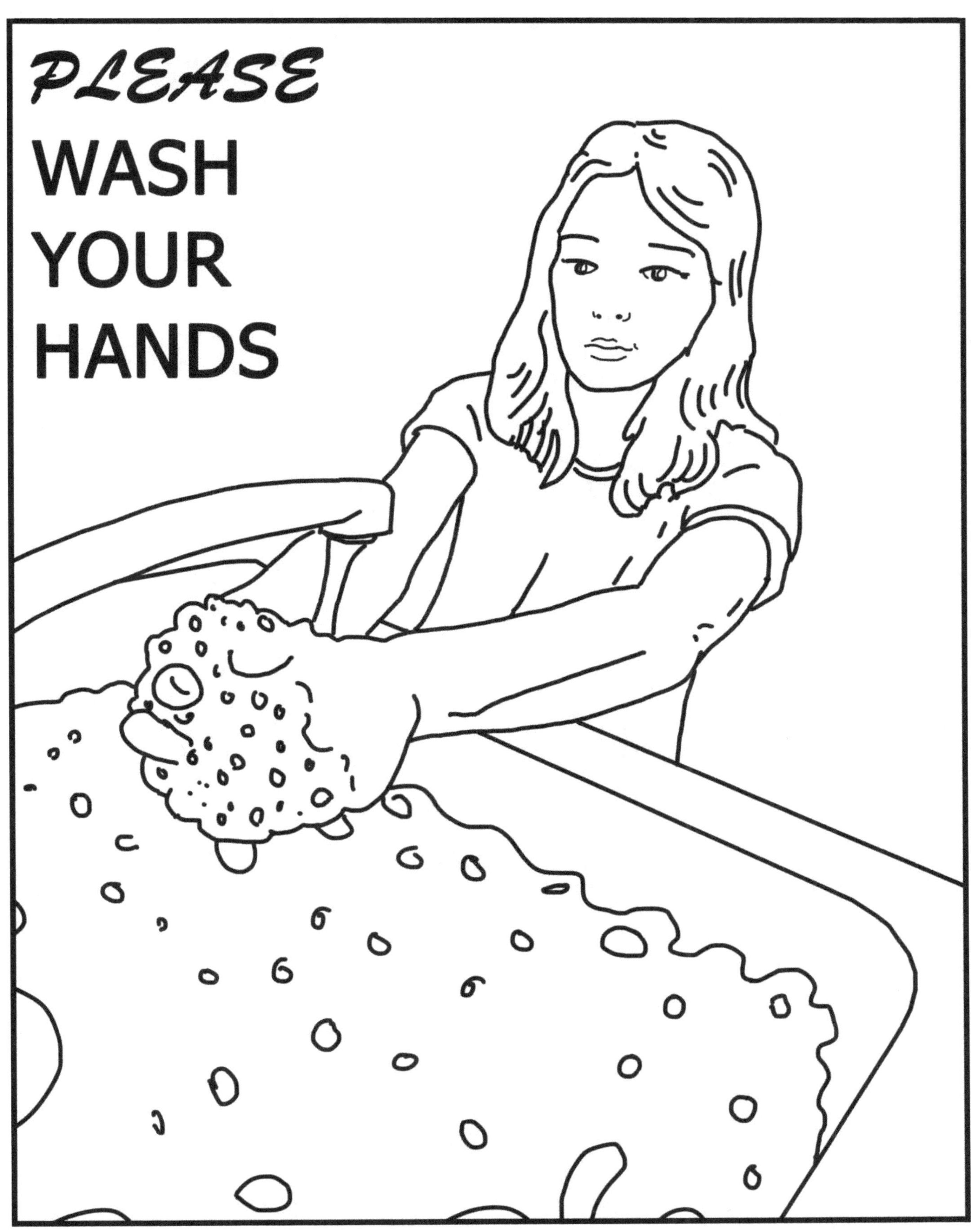

PLEASE
WASH
YOUR
HANDS

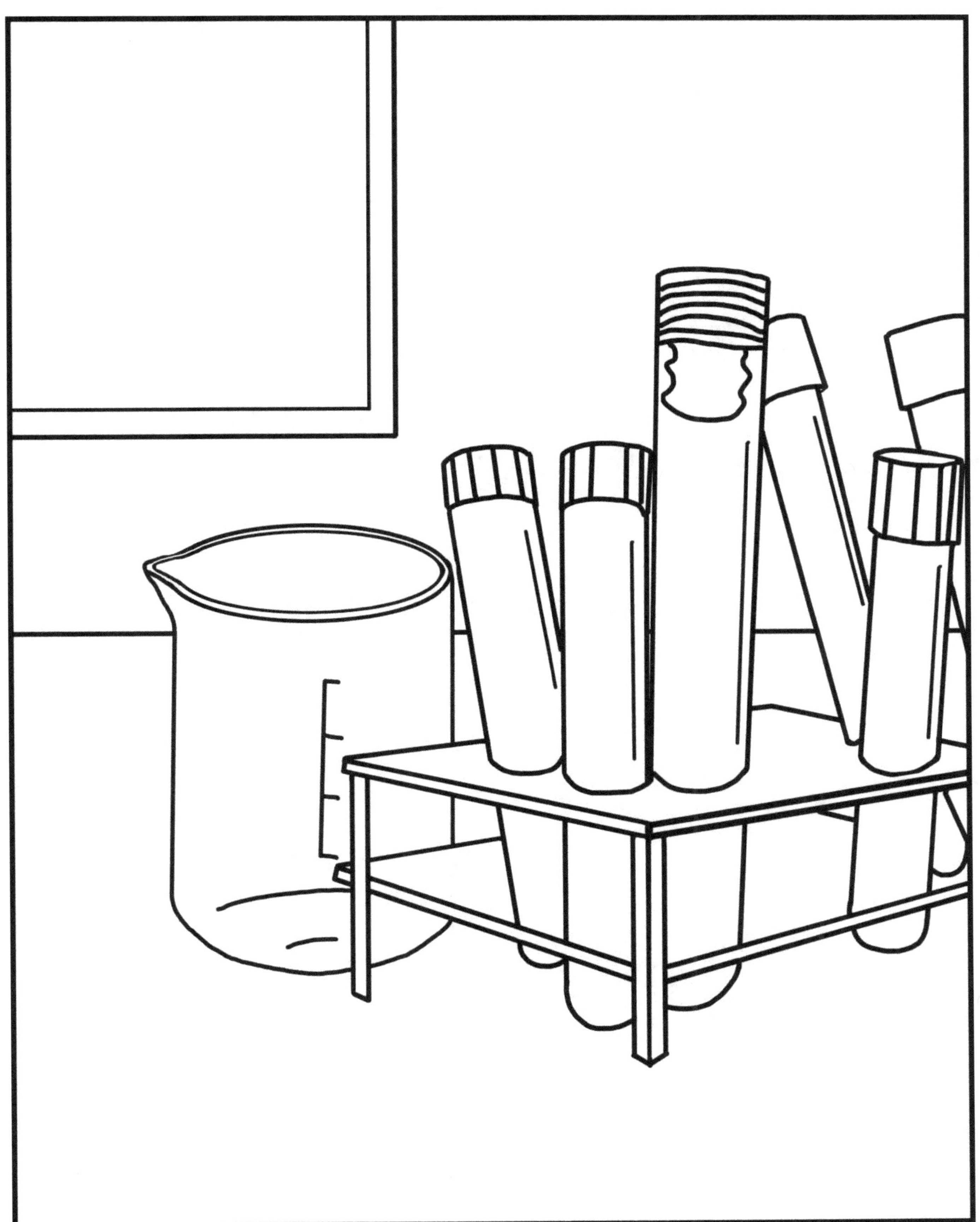

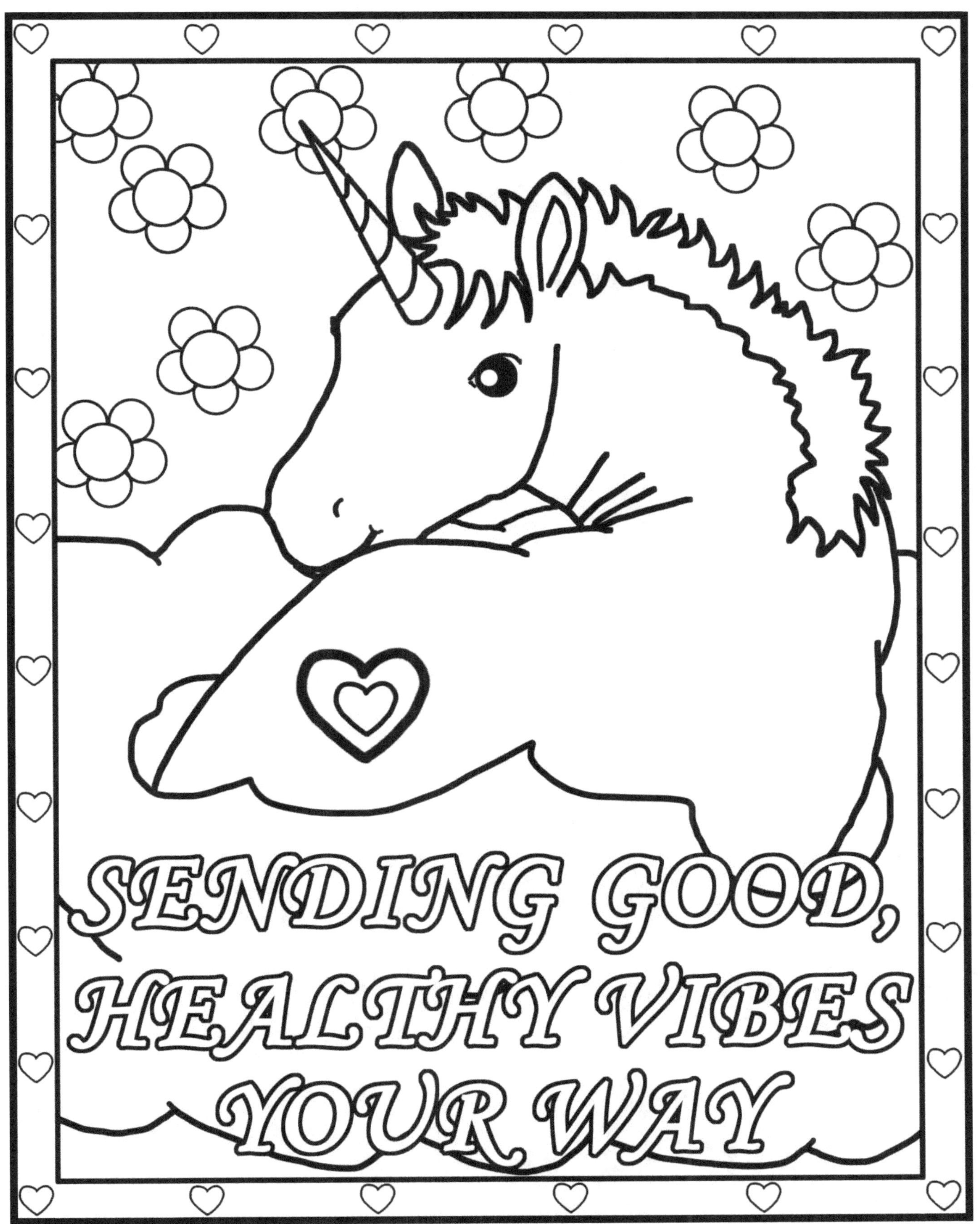

SENDING GOOD,
HEALTHY VIBES
YOUR WAY

# Bless you!

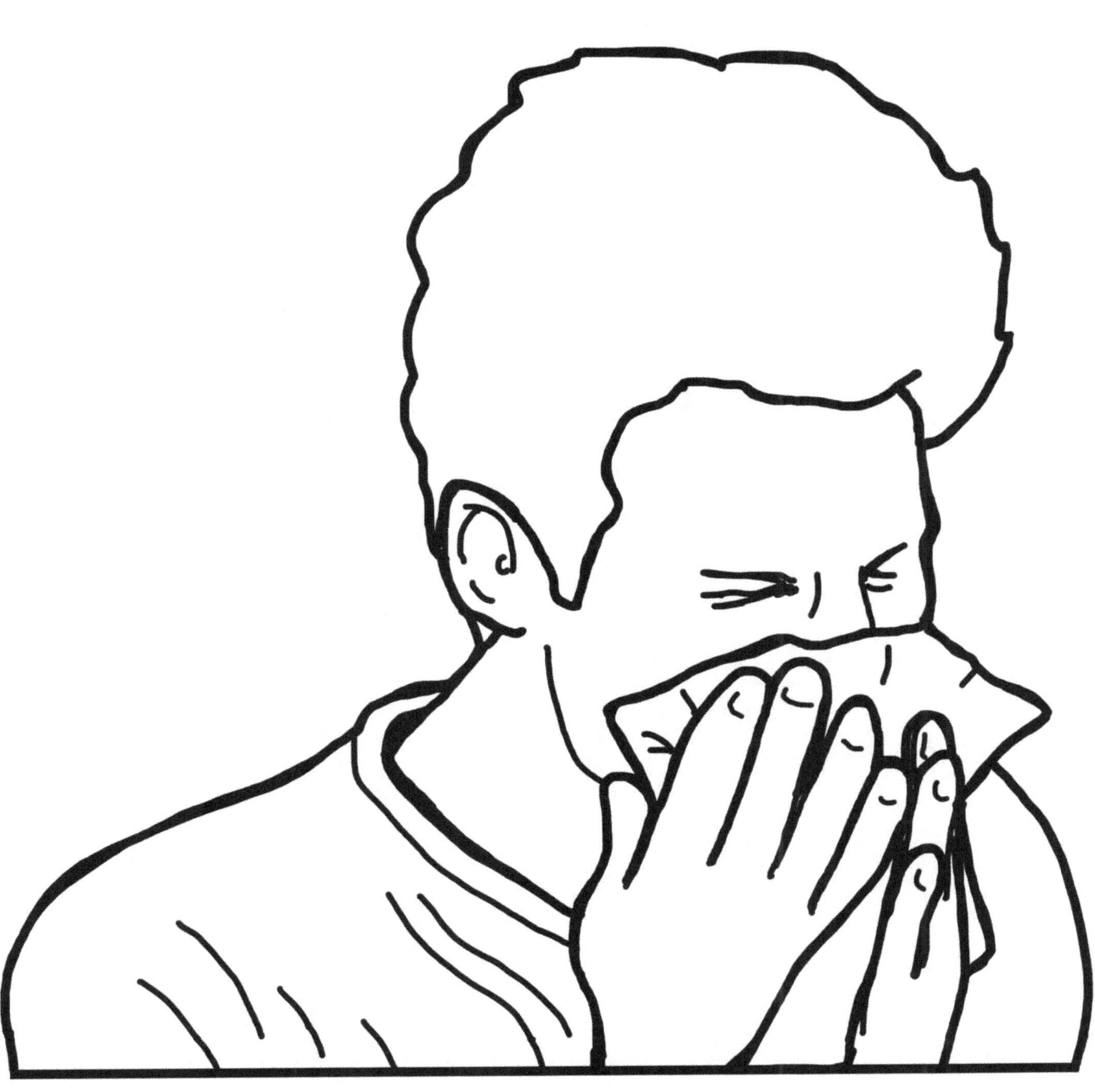

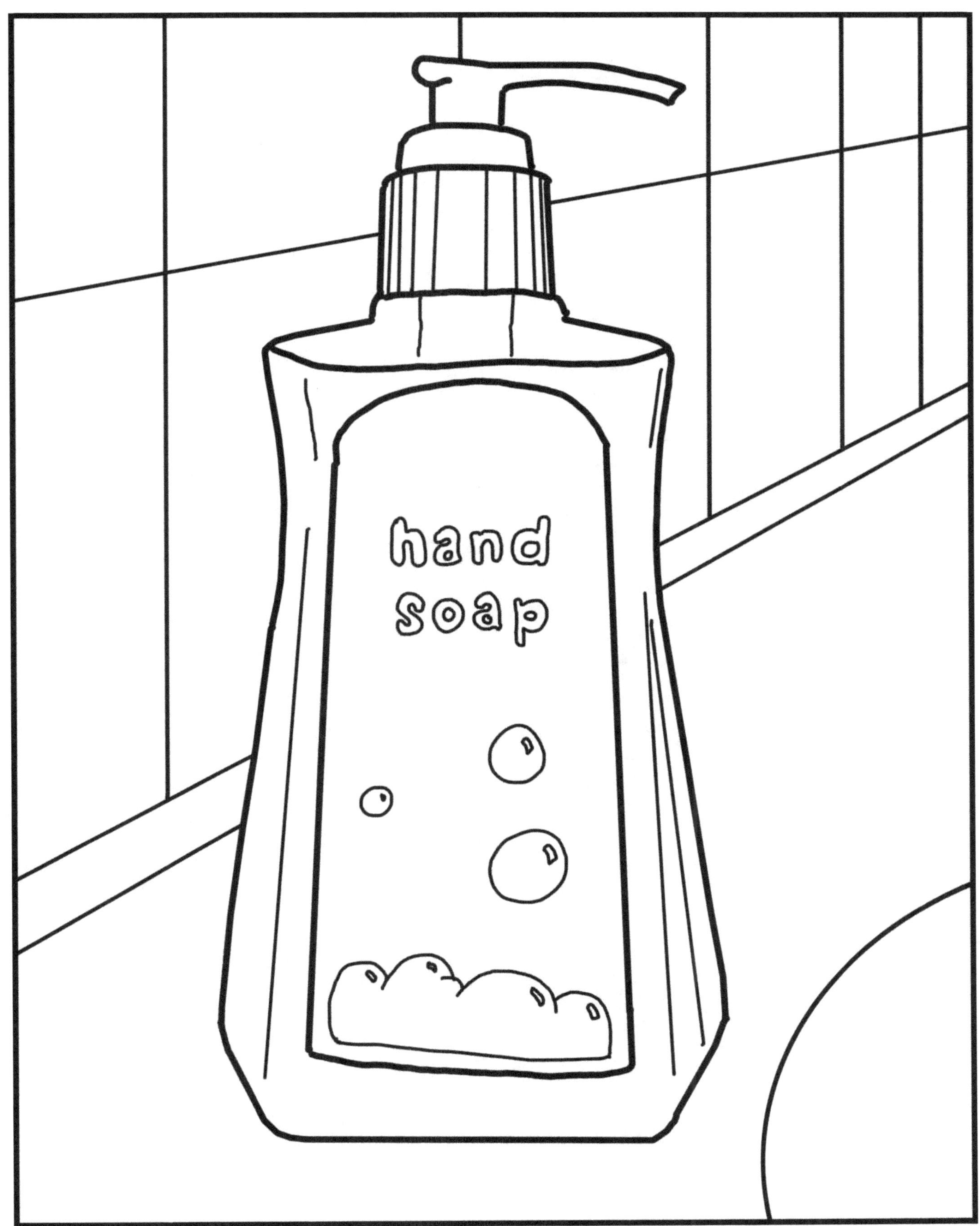
hand
soap

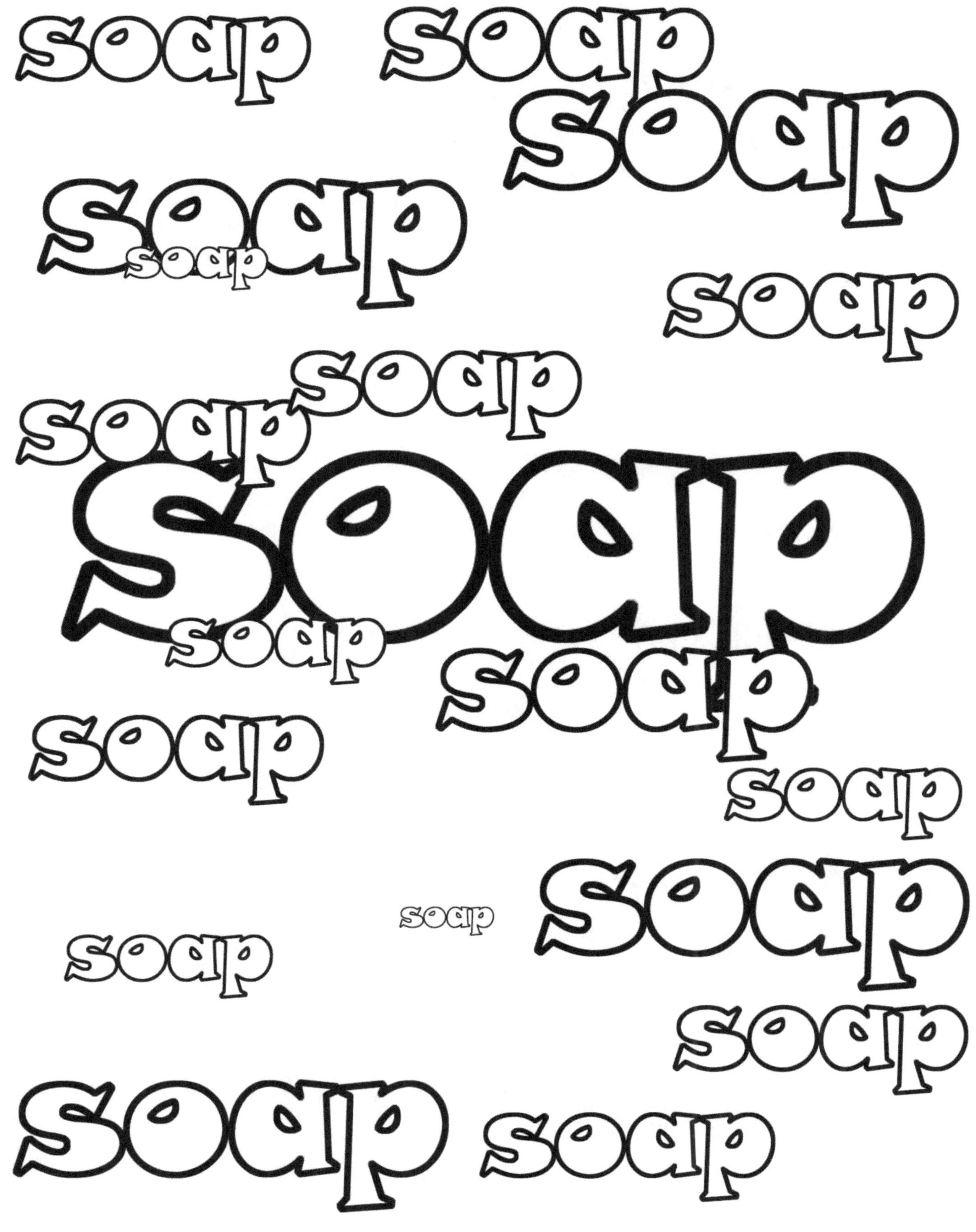

soap
soap
soap
soap
soap
soap
soap
soap
soap
soap
soap
soap
soap
soap
soap
soap
soap

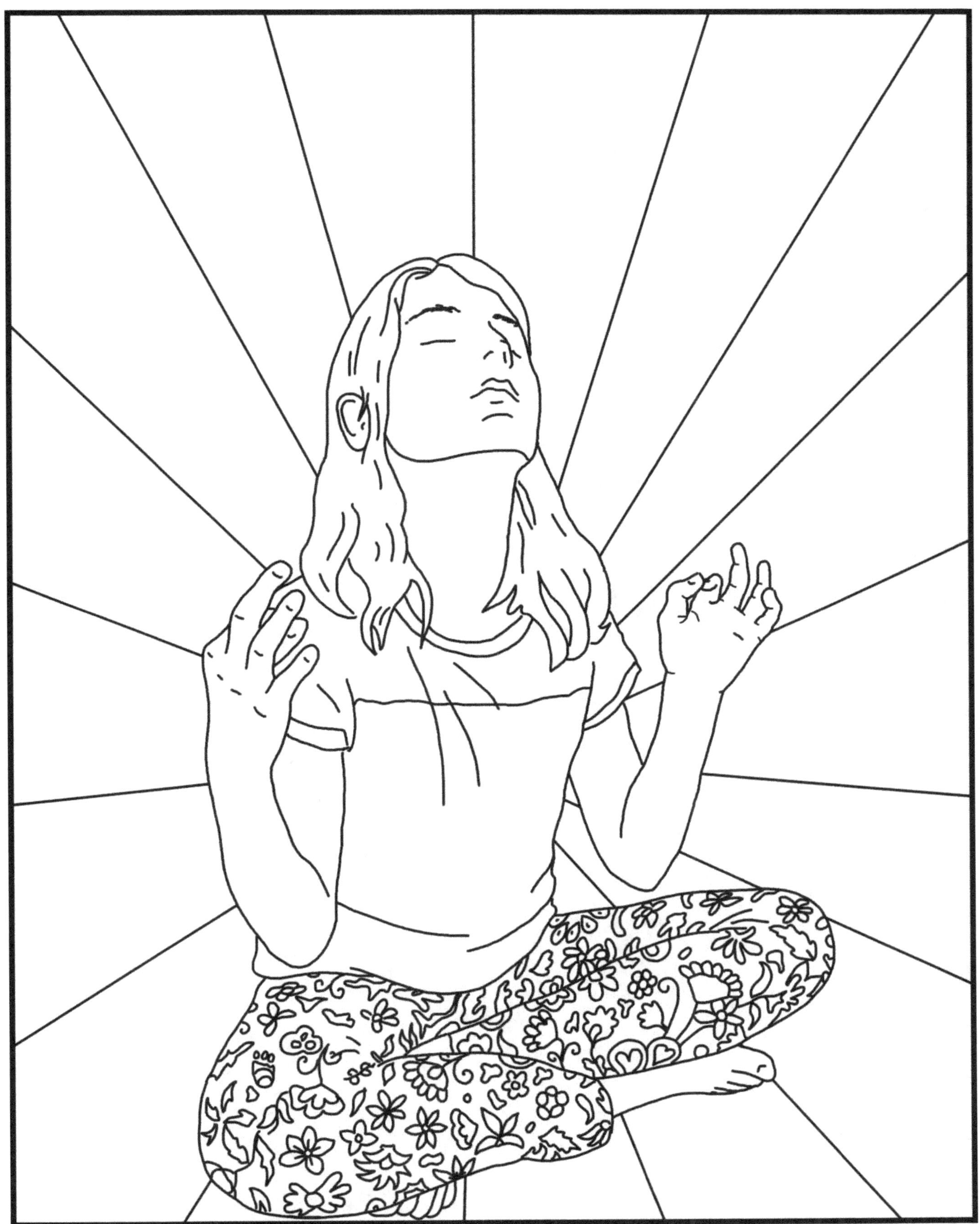

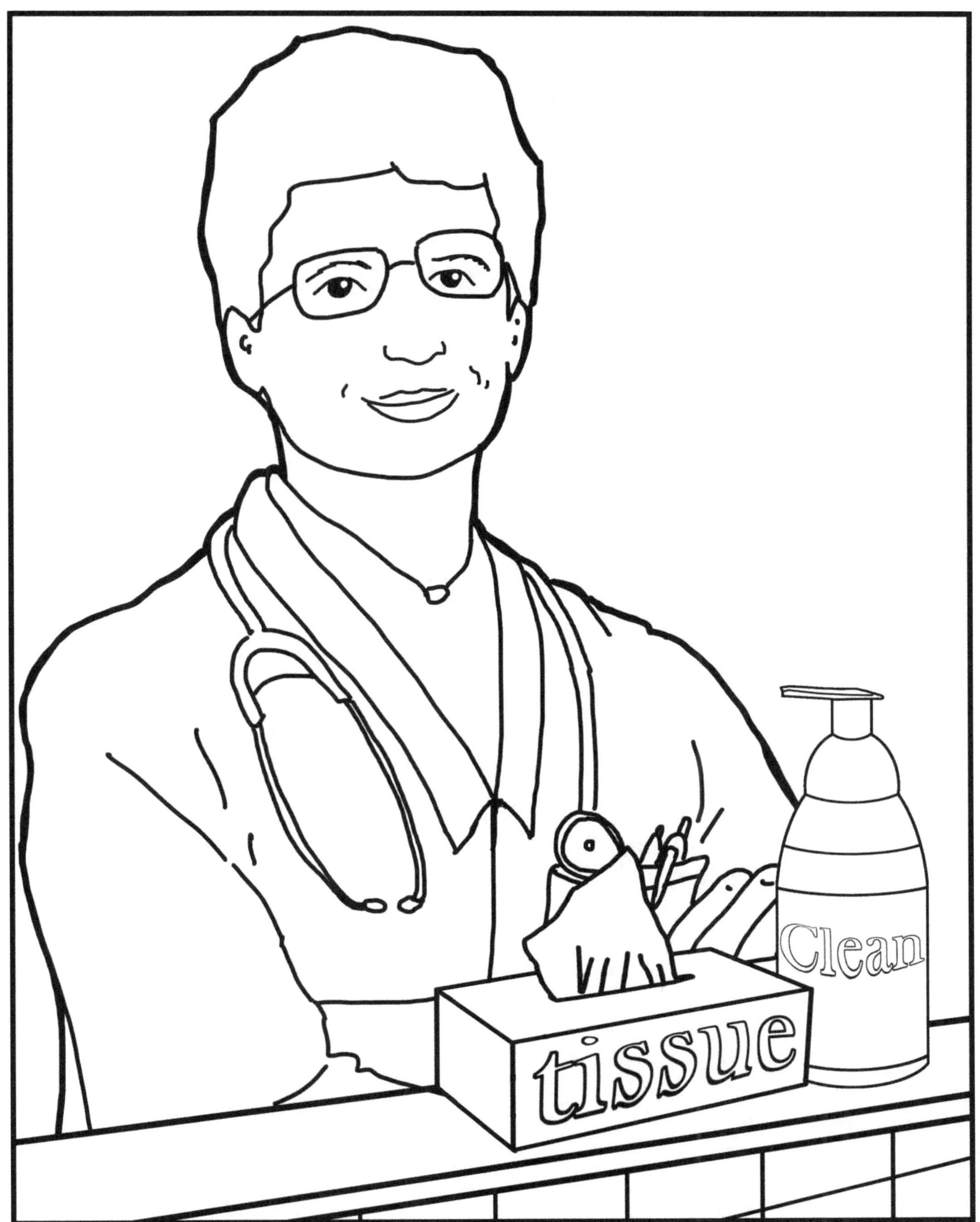

tissue
Clean

HUGS AND KISSES, GET WELL WISHES

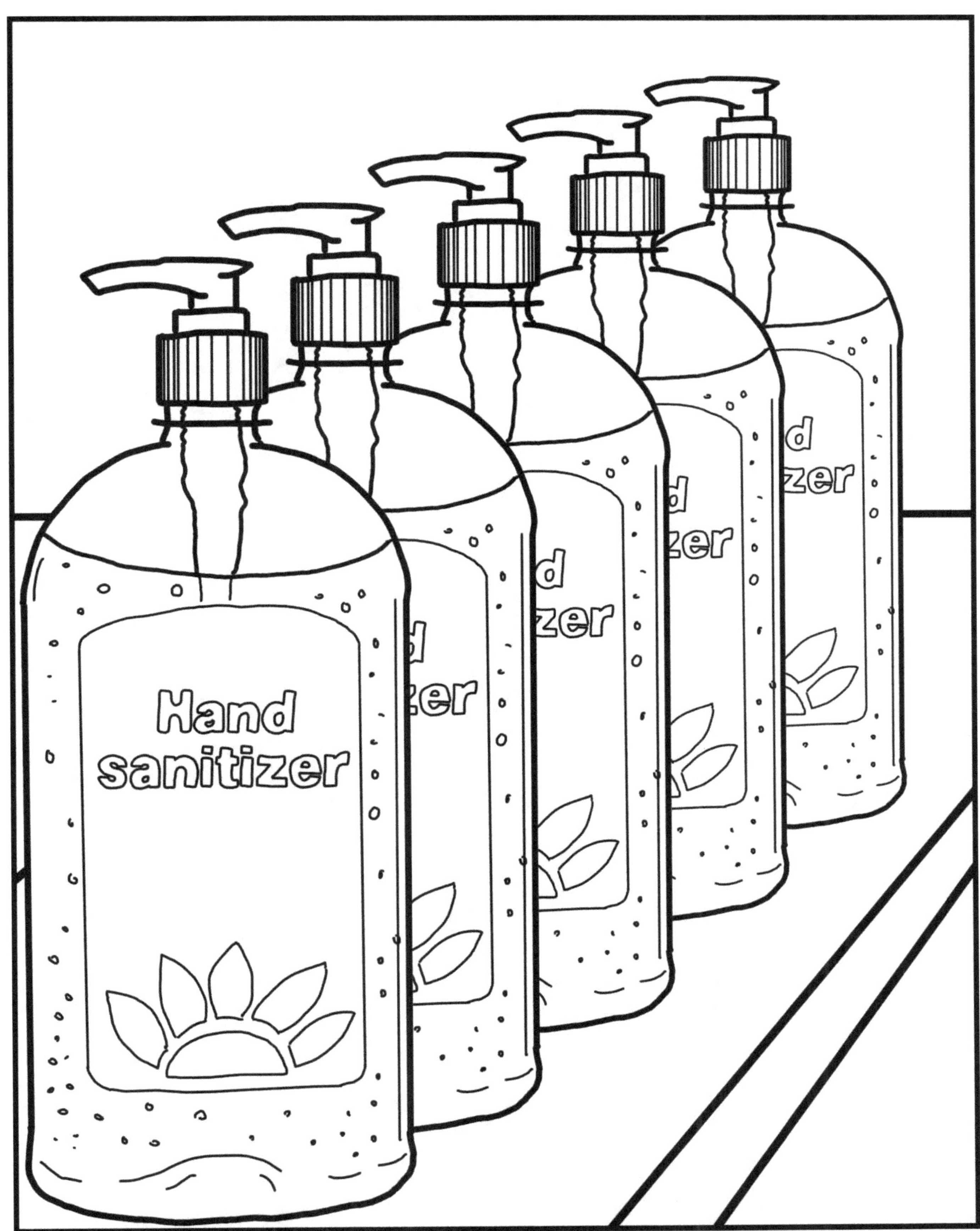

Hand
sanitizer

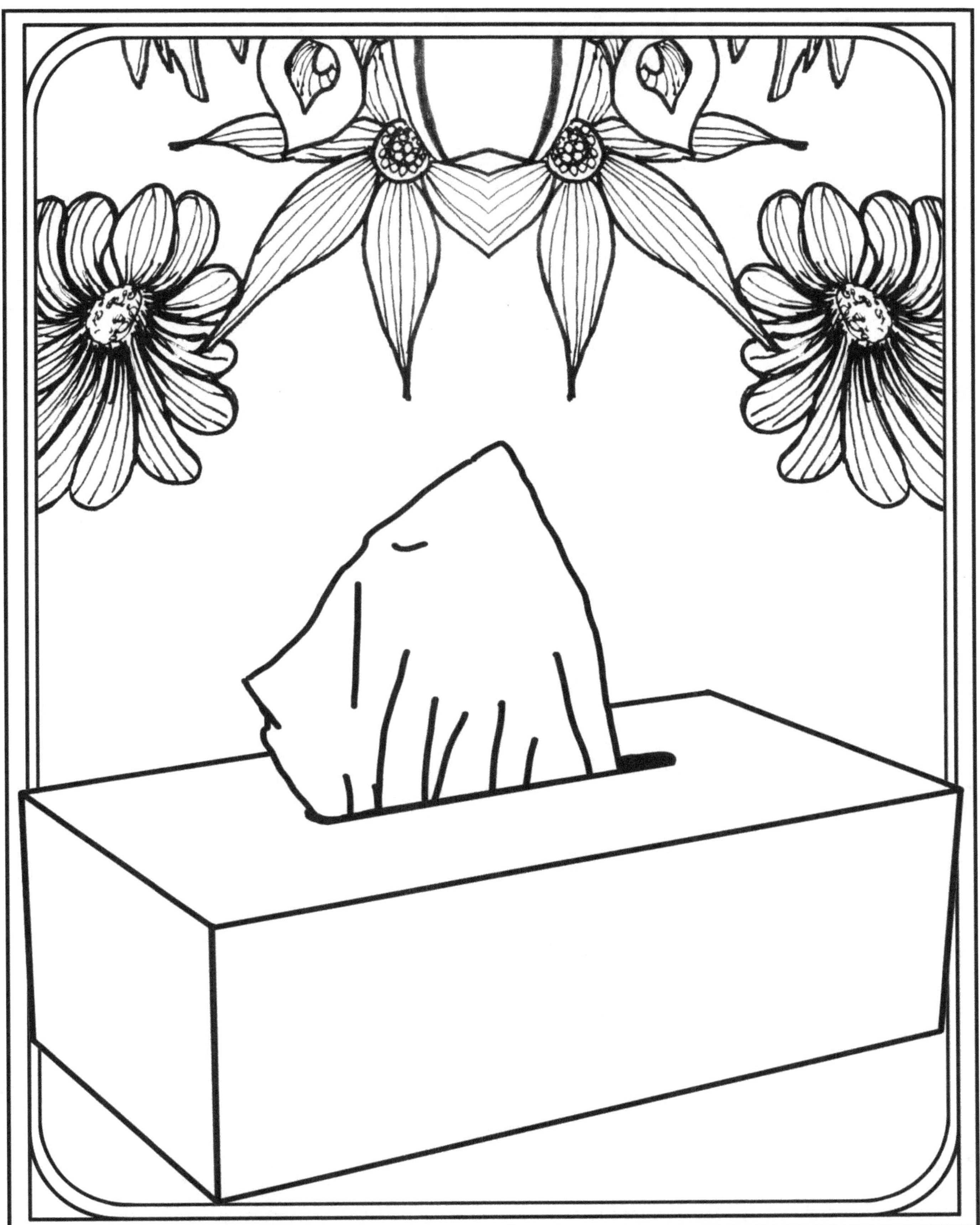

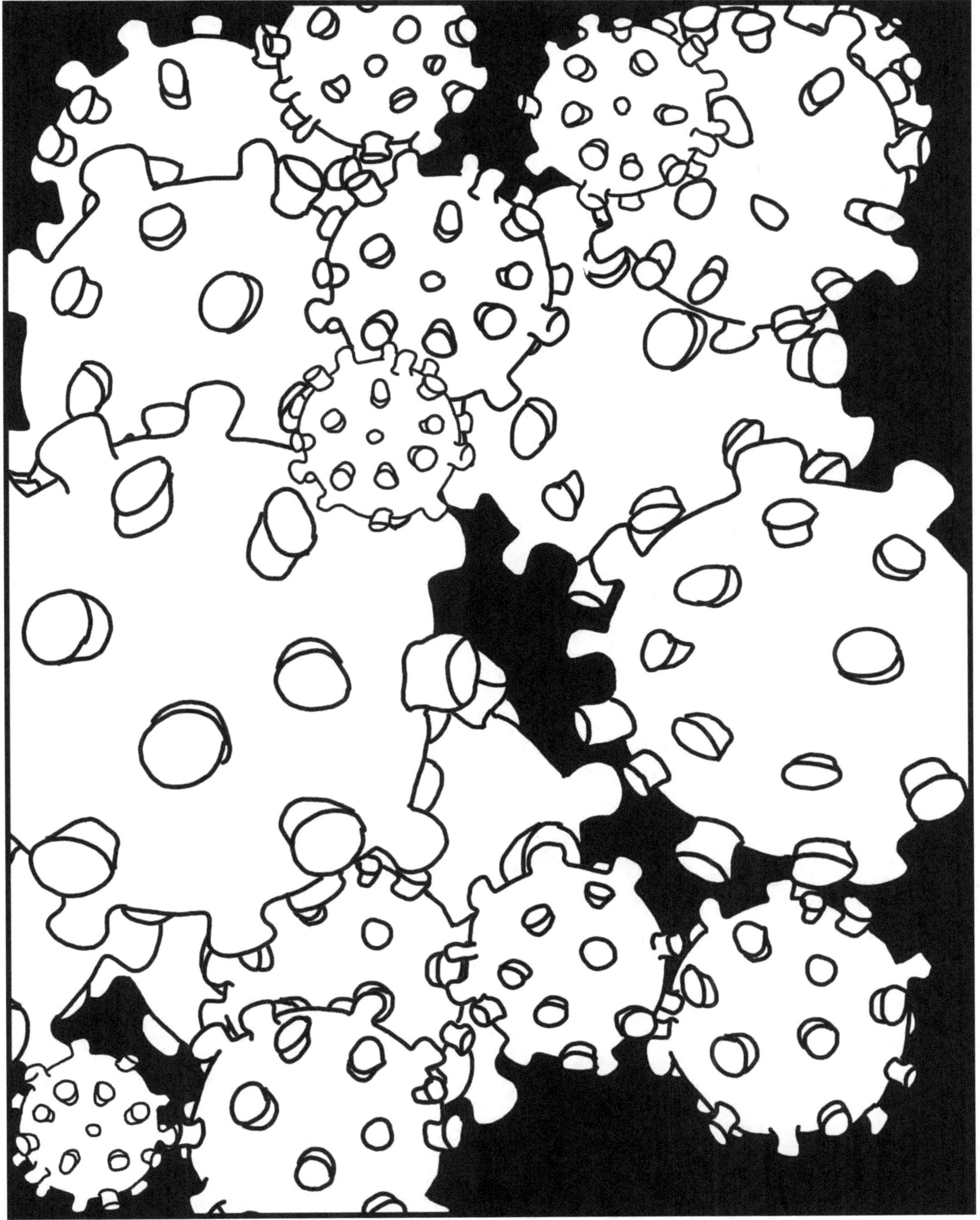

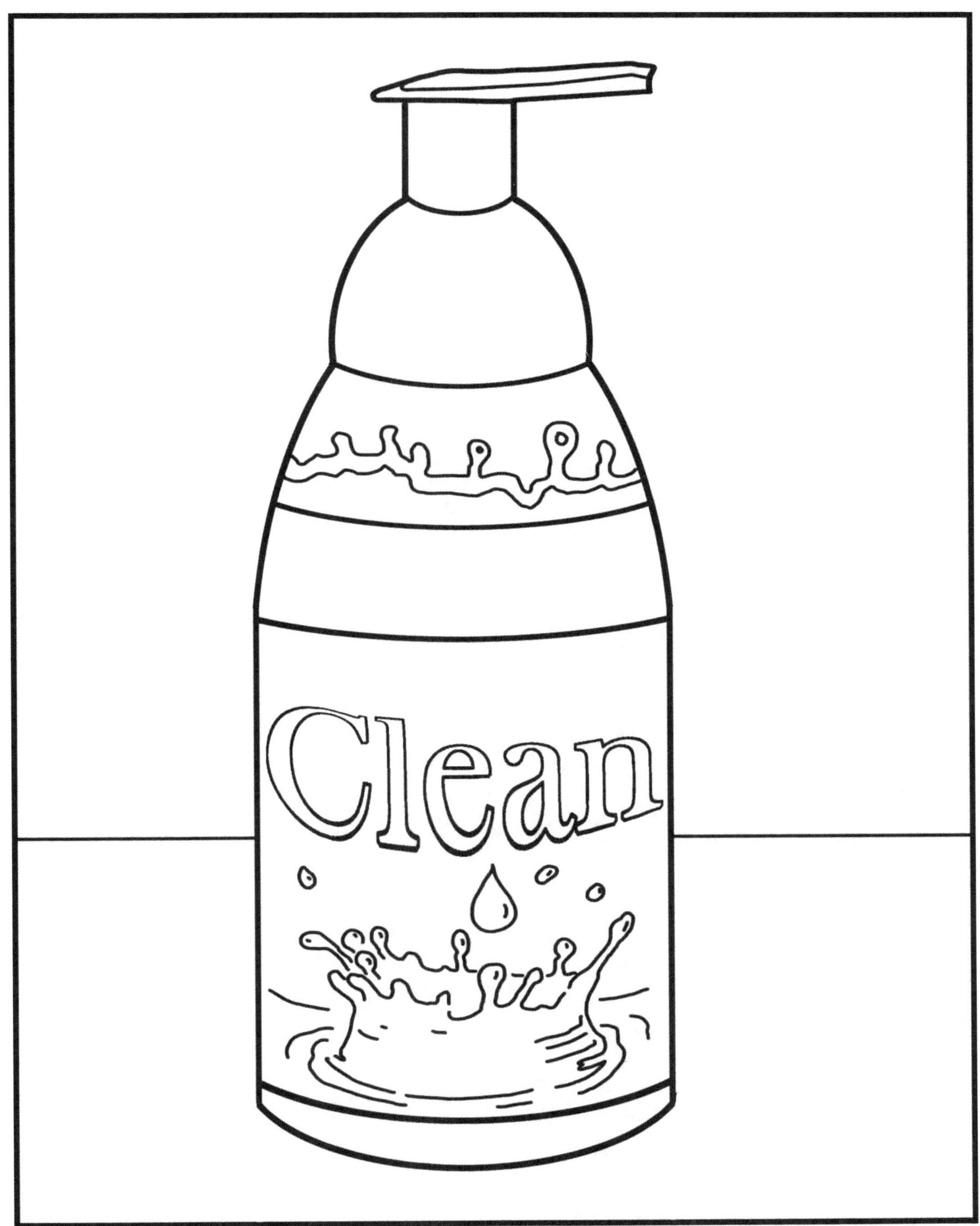
Clean

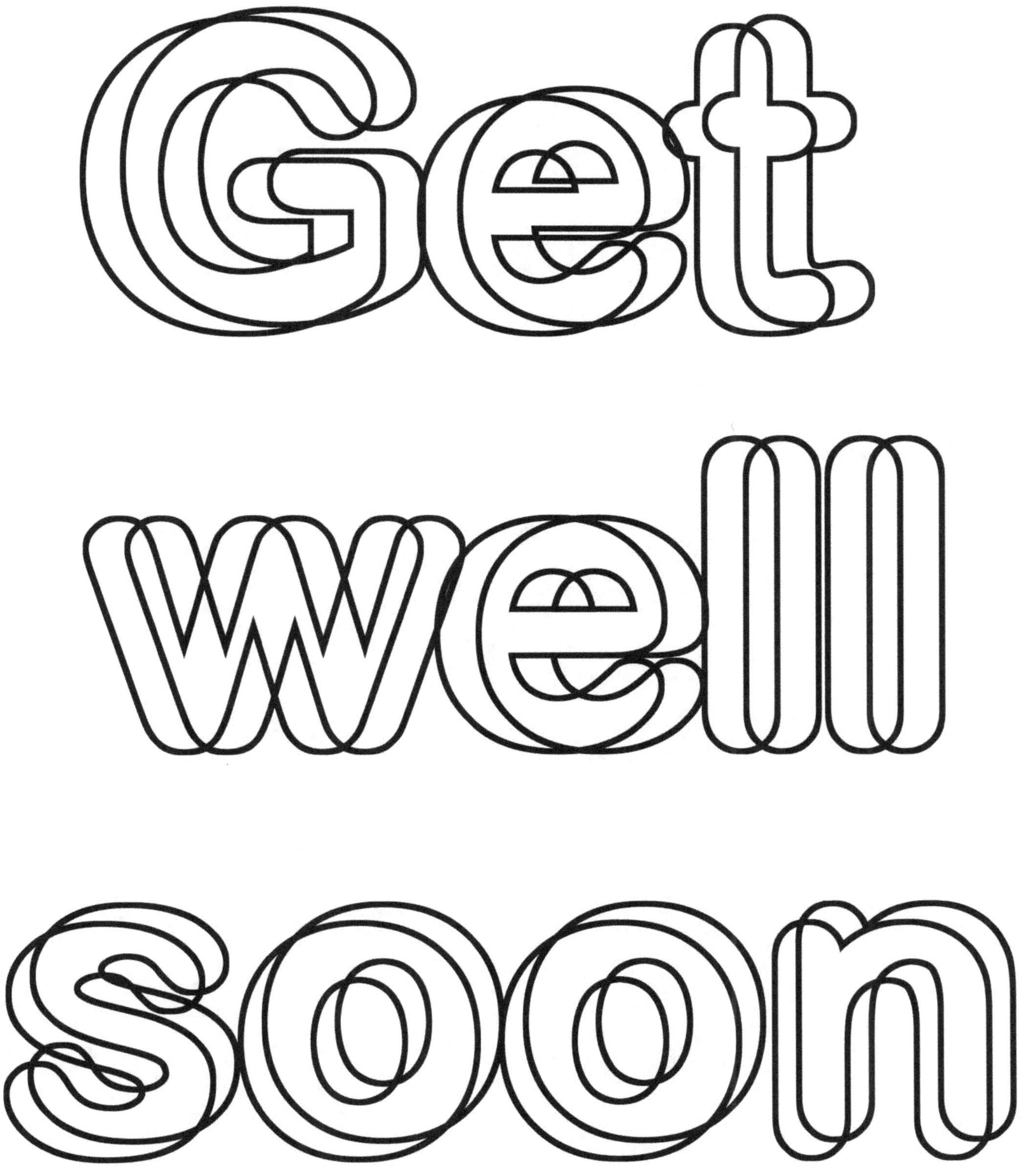
Get well soon

# Strength

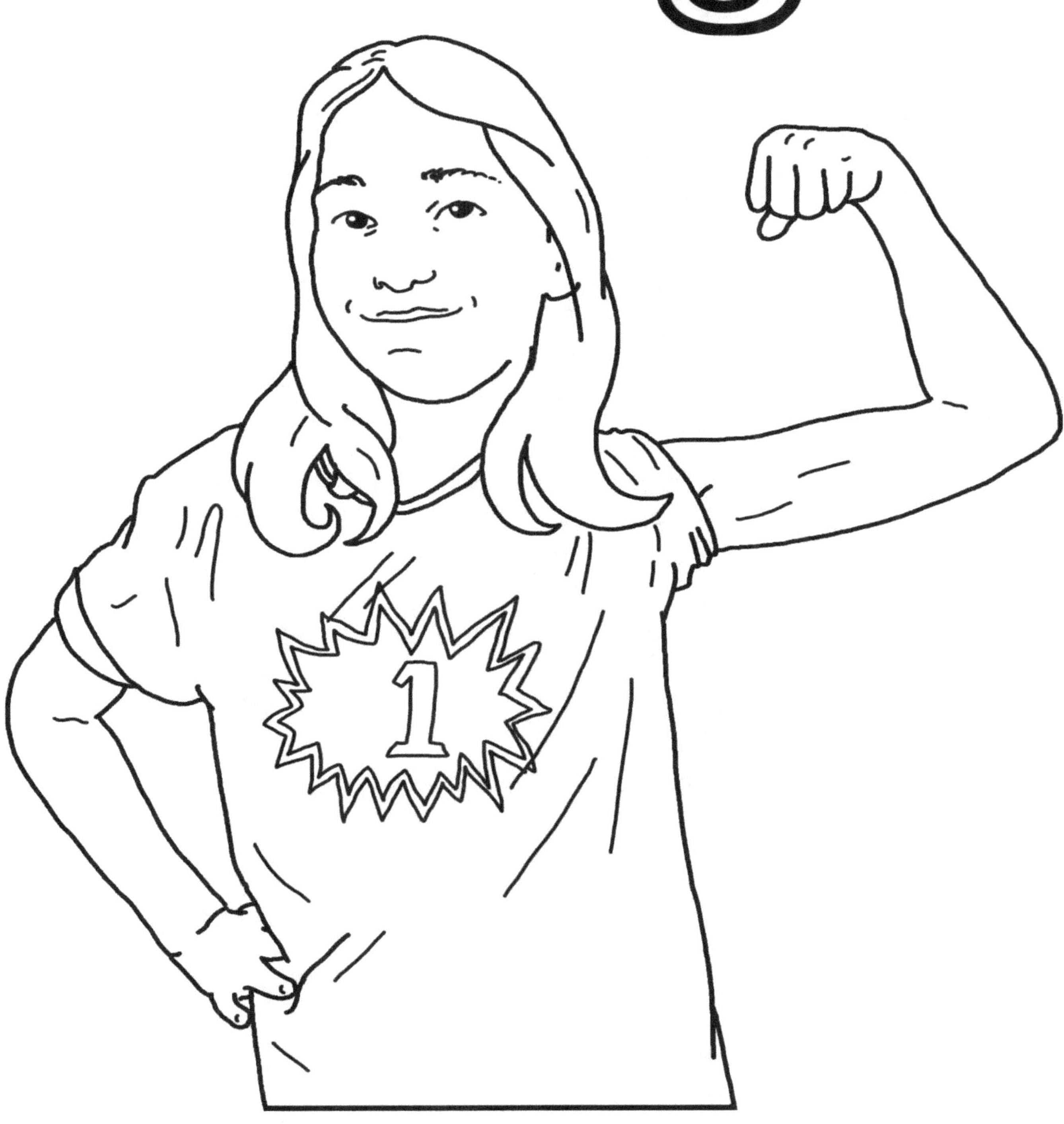

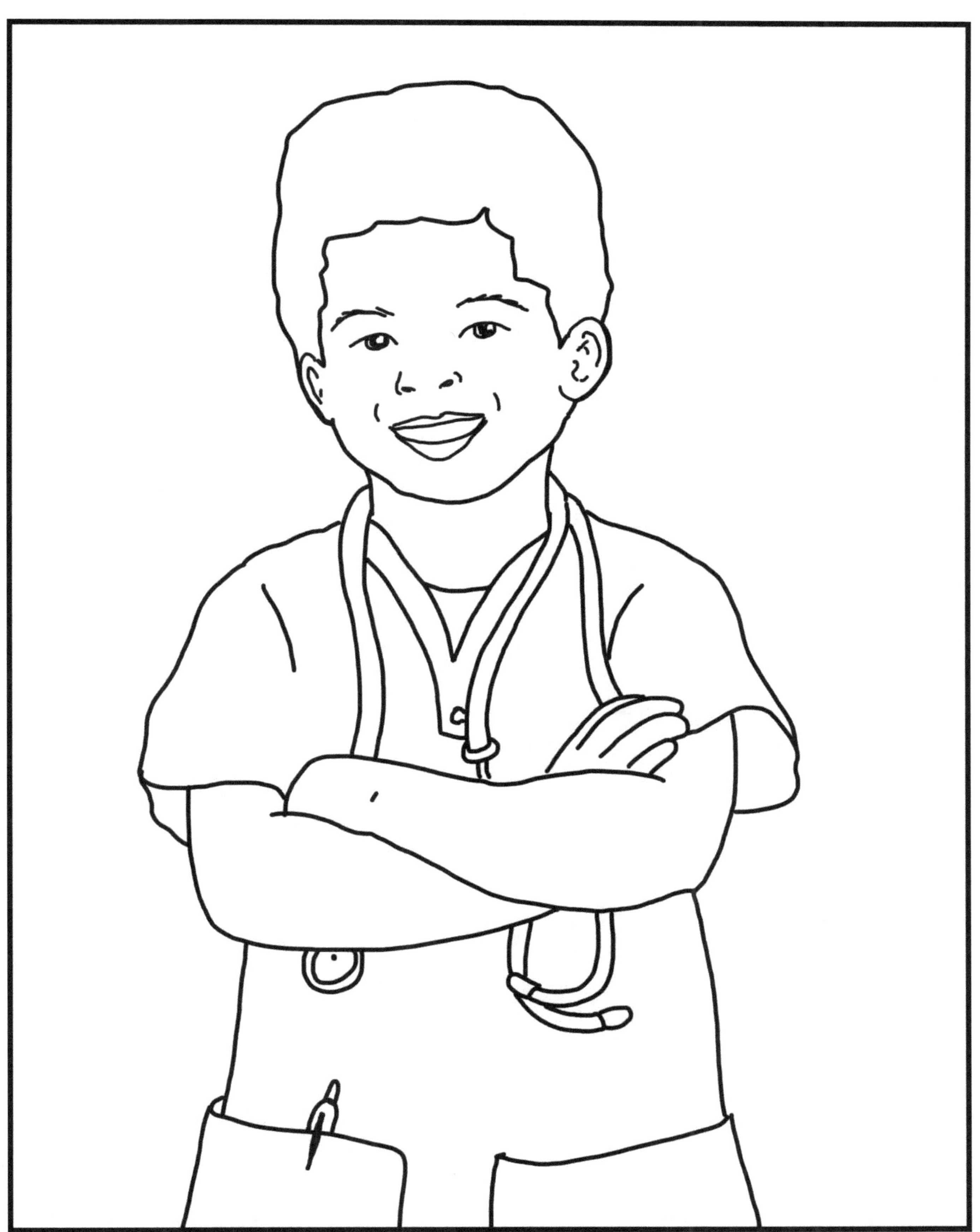

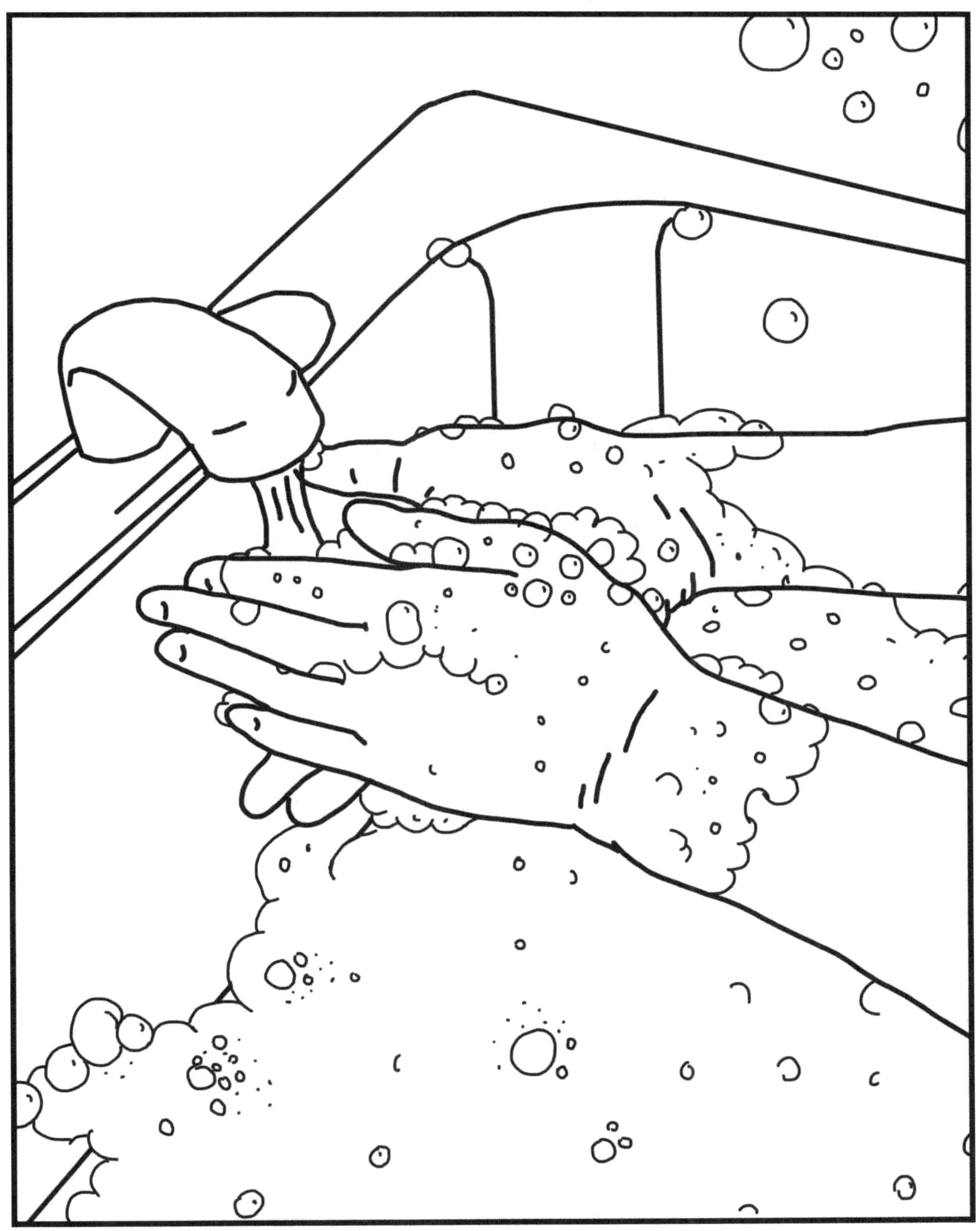

Sending you
well wishes
for your
quick recovery
and good health

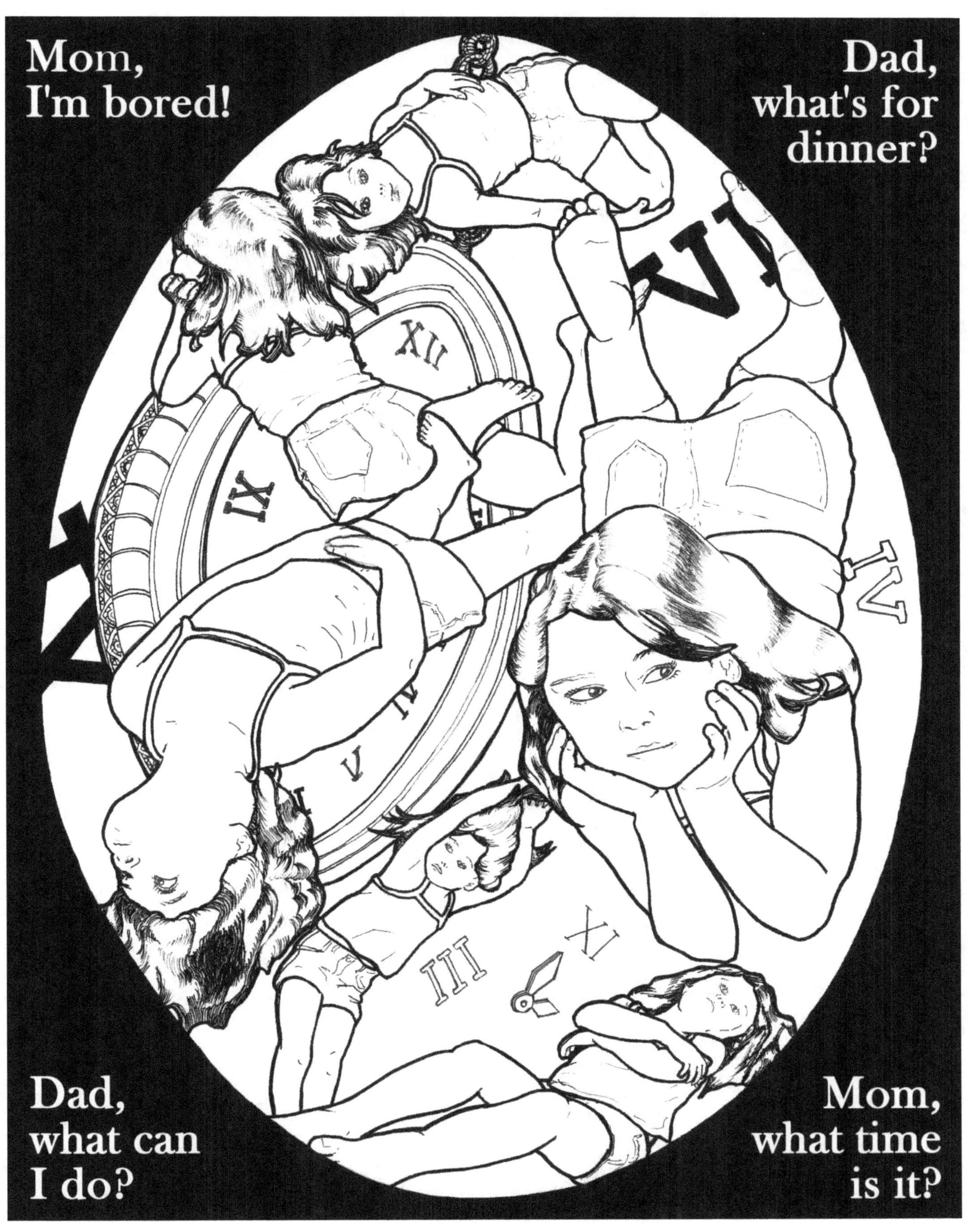

Mom,
I'm bored!
Dad,
what's for
dinner?
Dad,
what can
I do?
Mom,
what time
is it?

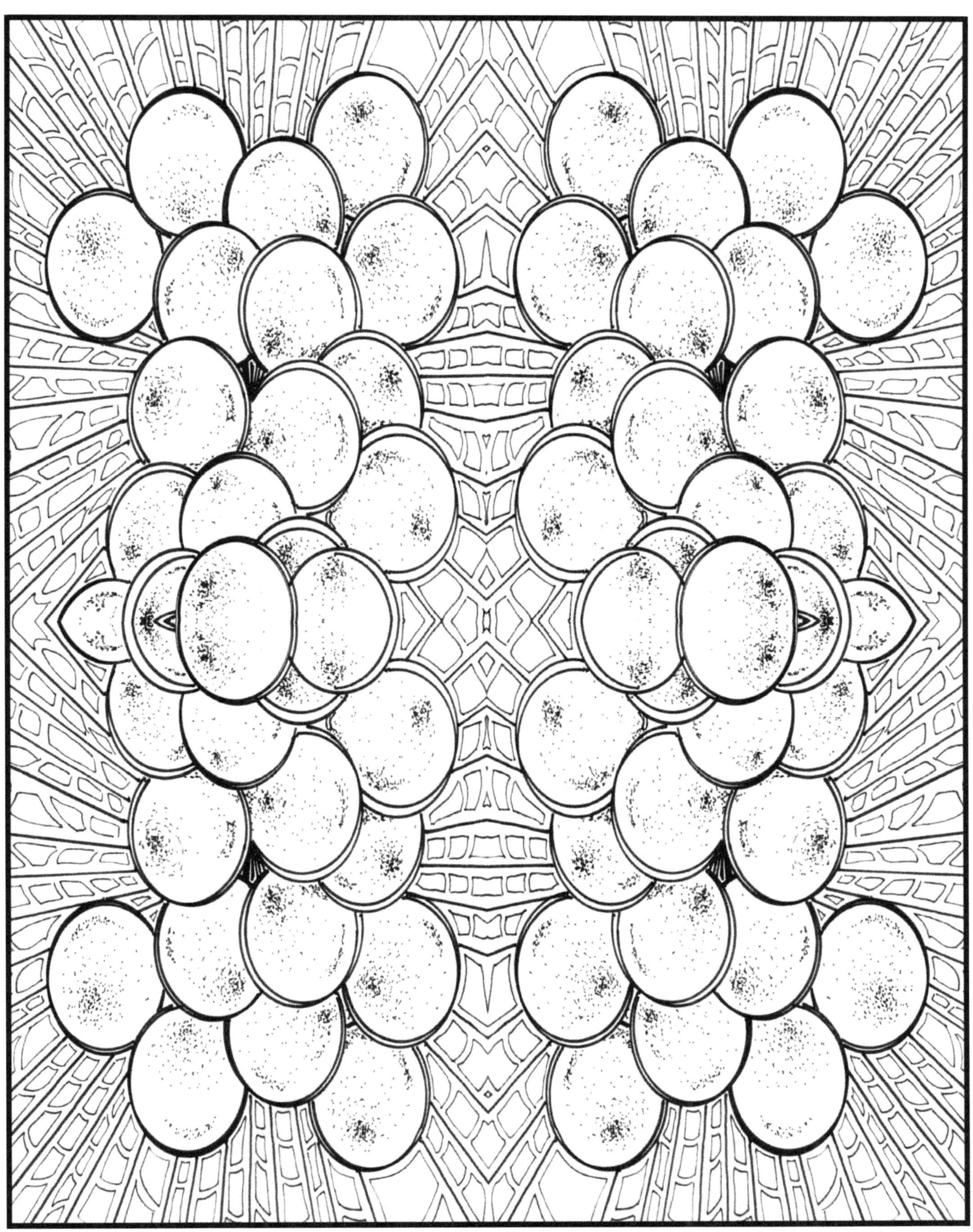

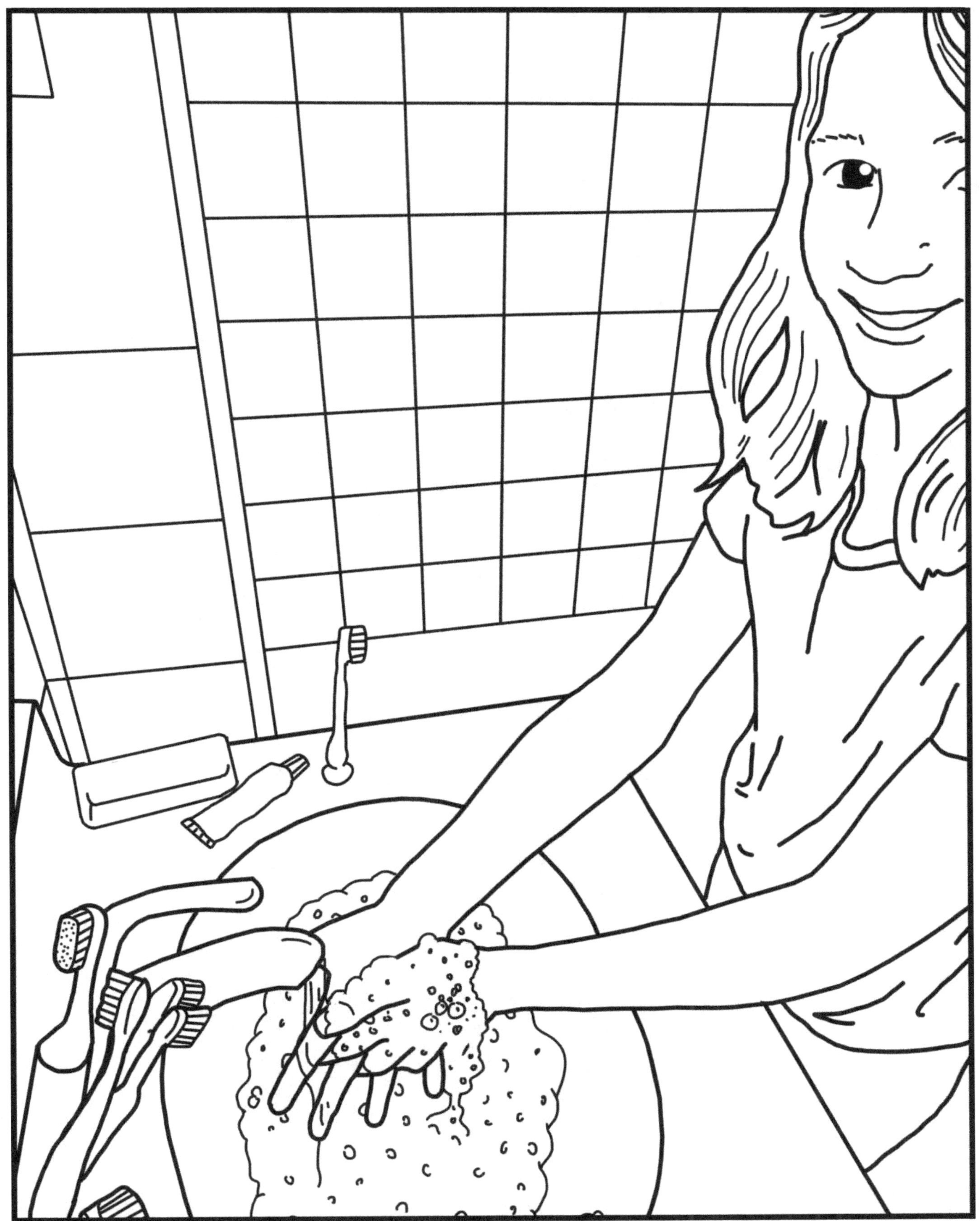

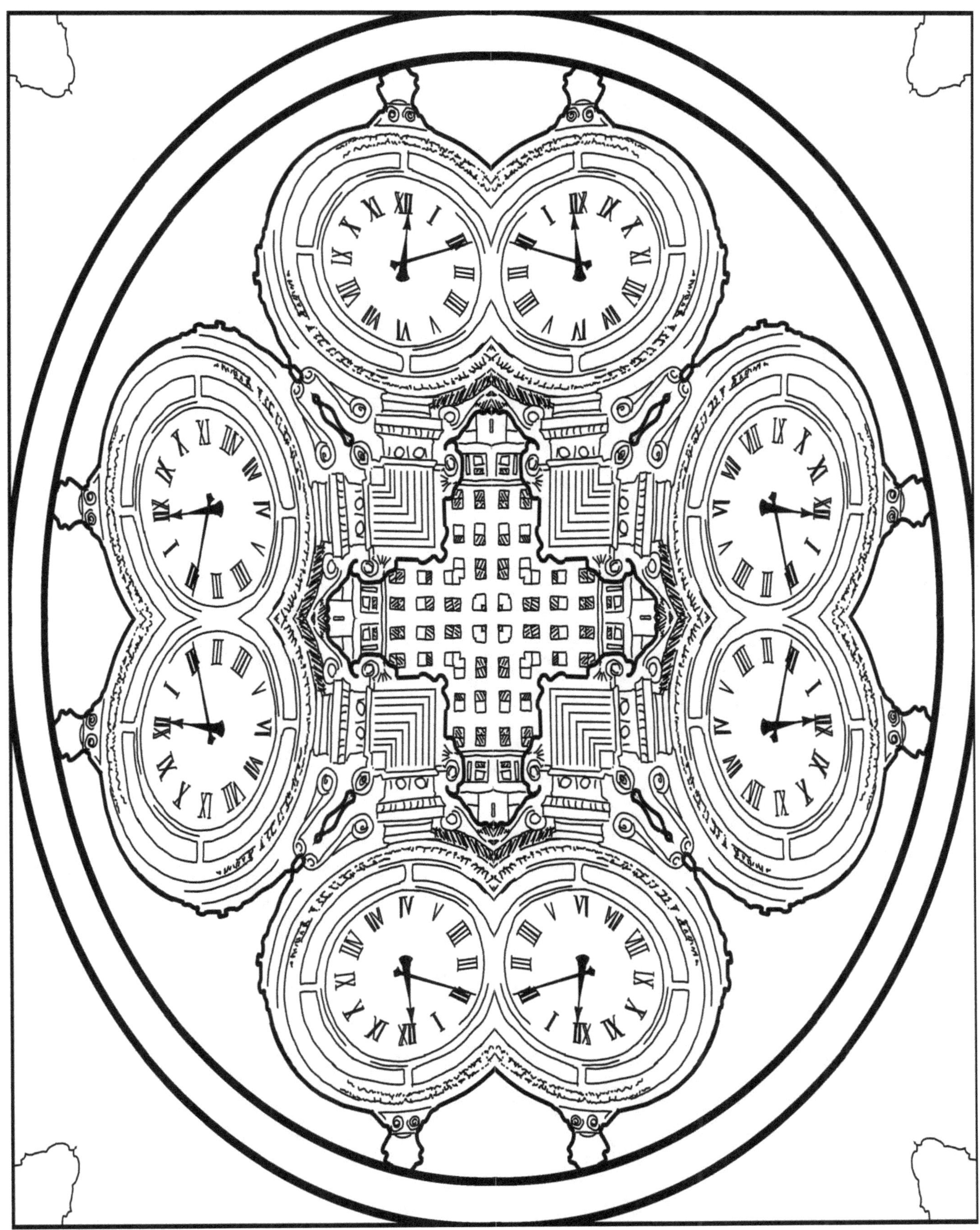

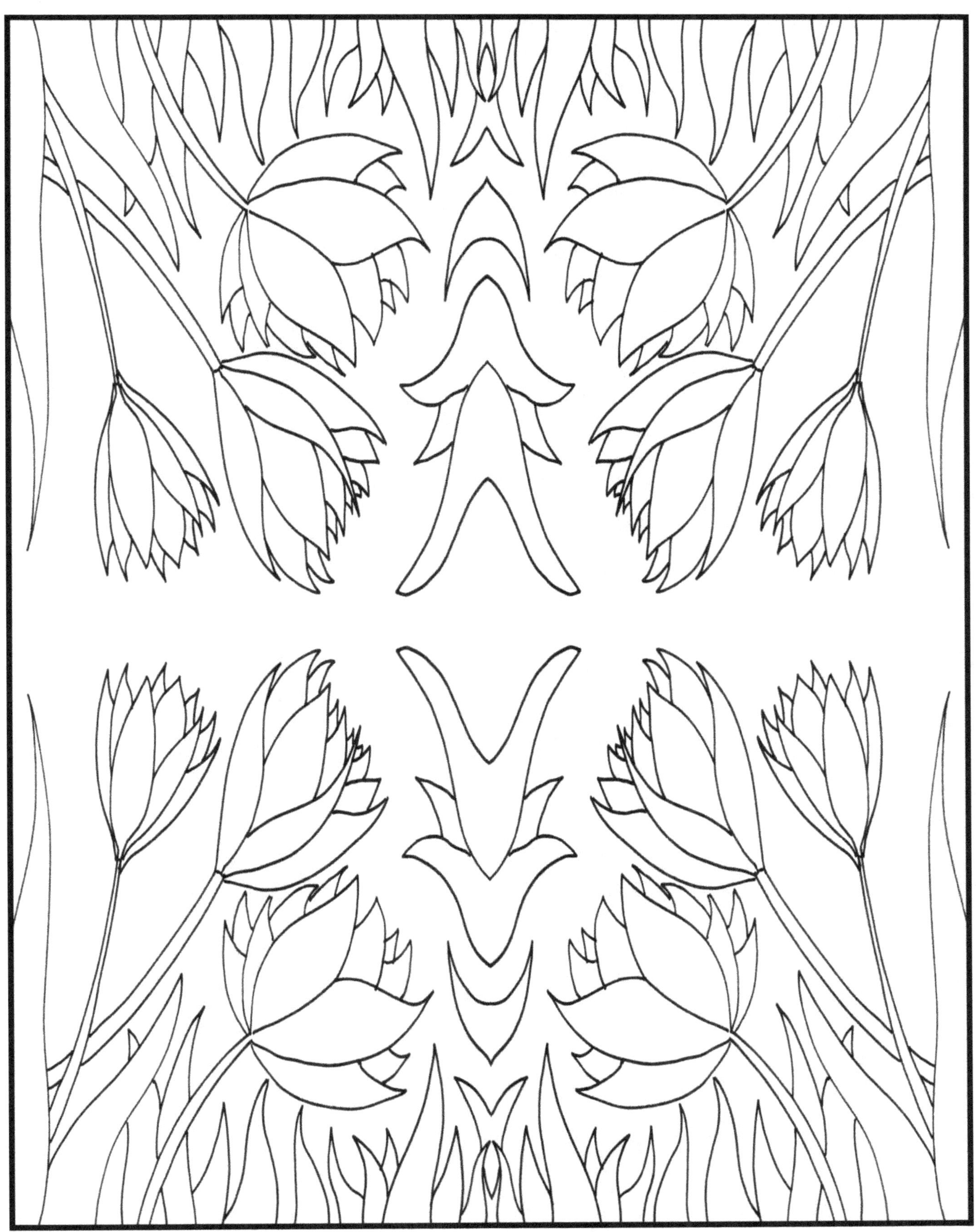

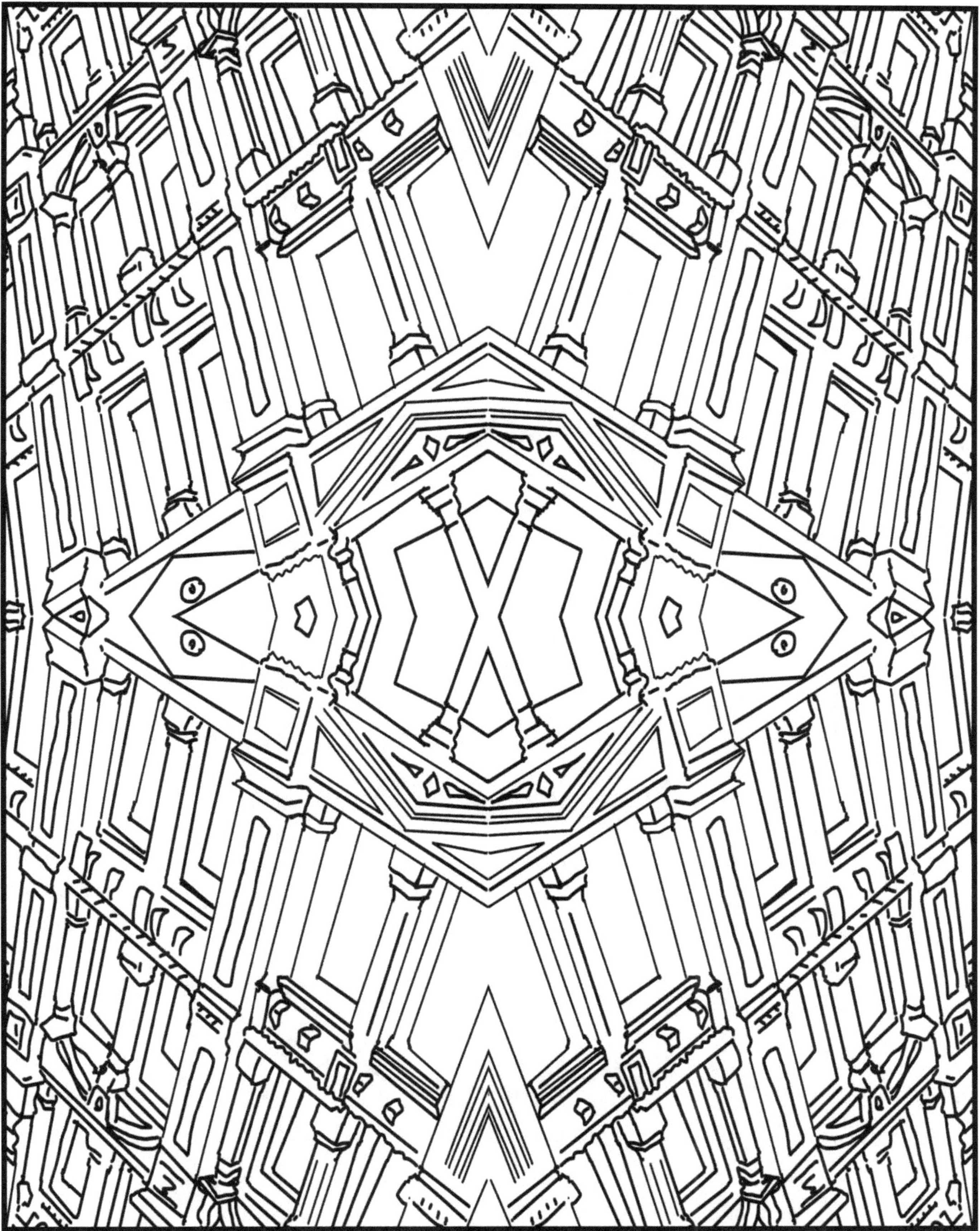

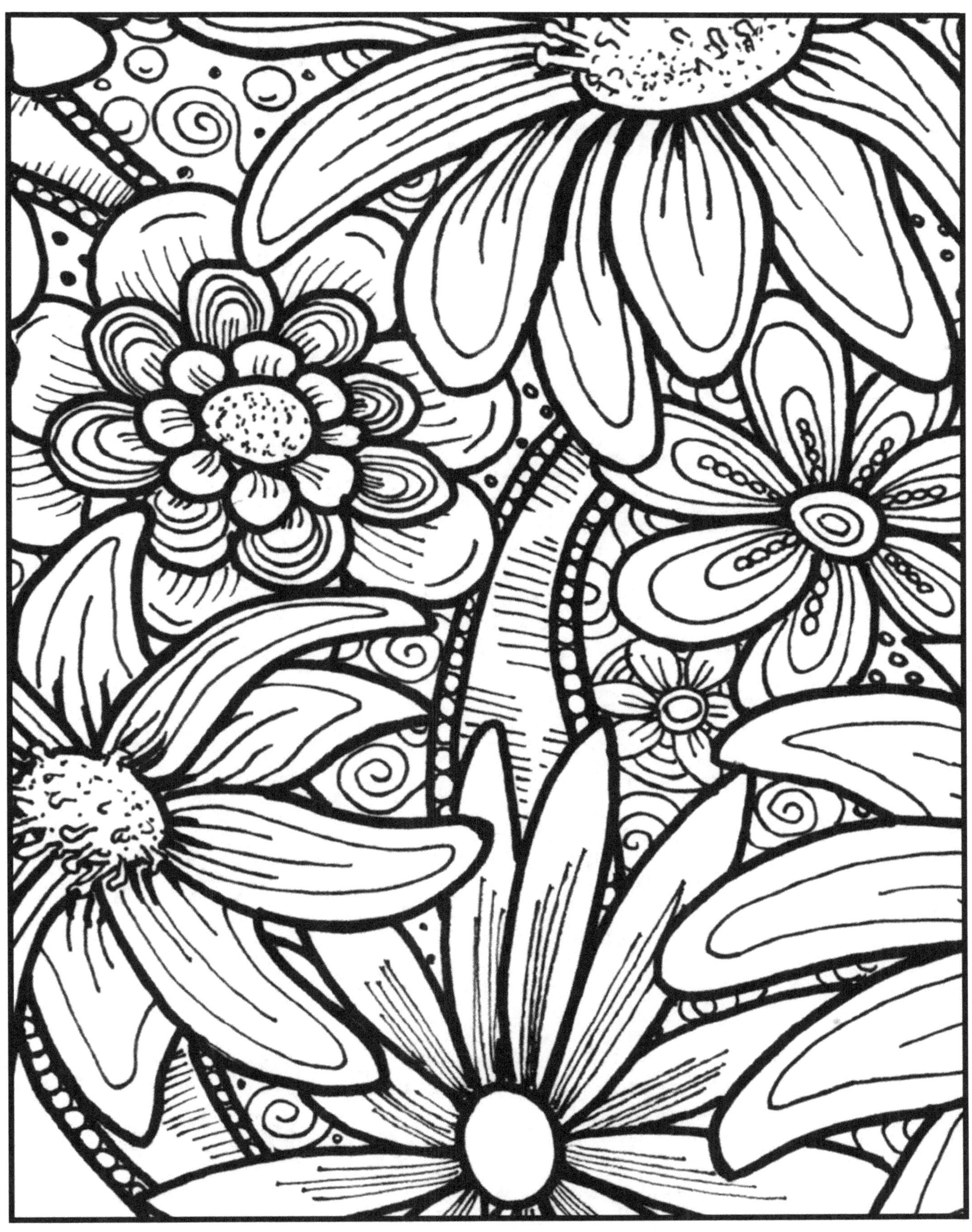

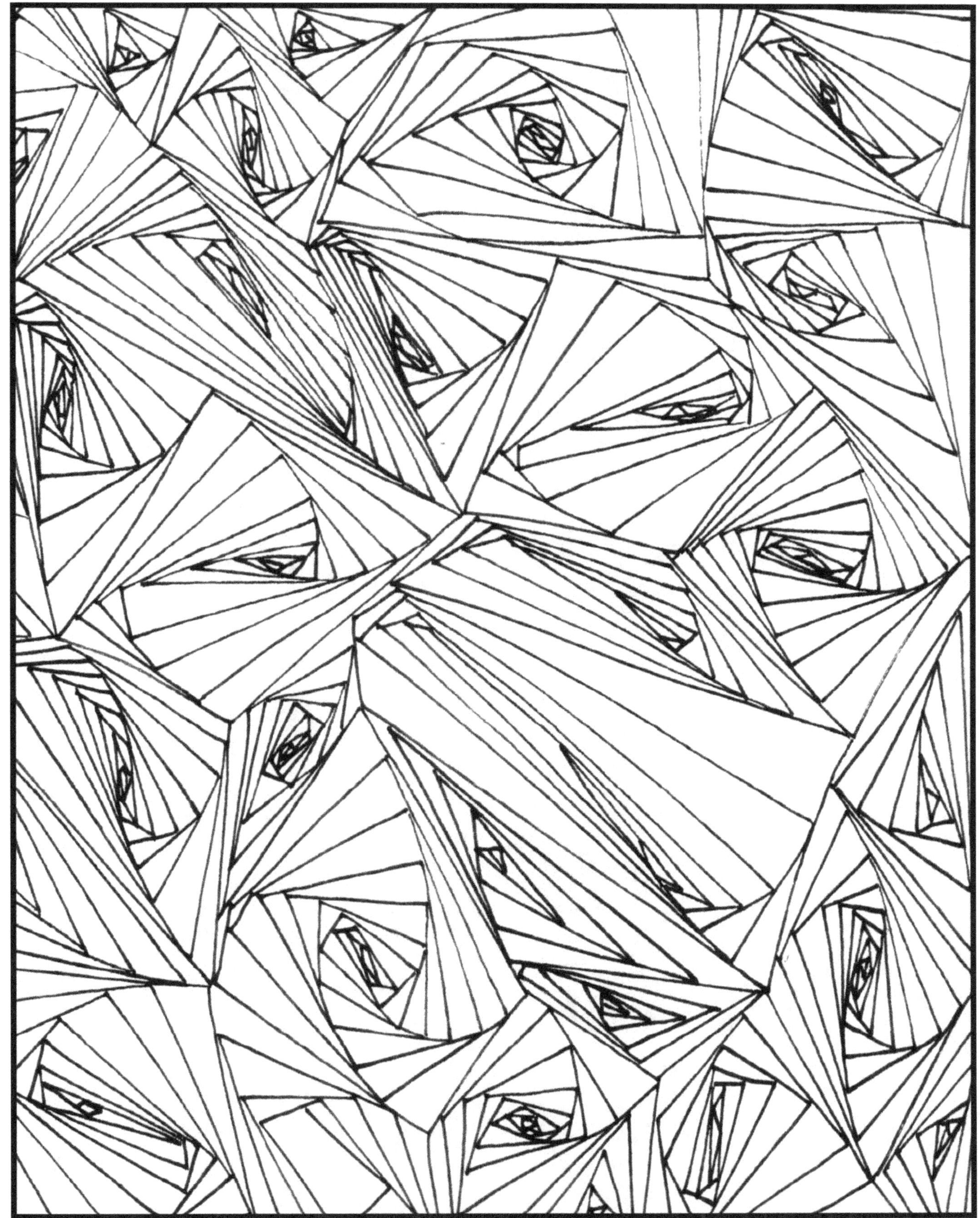

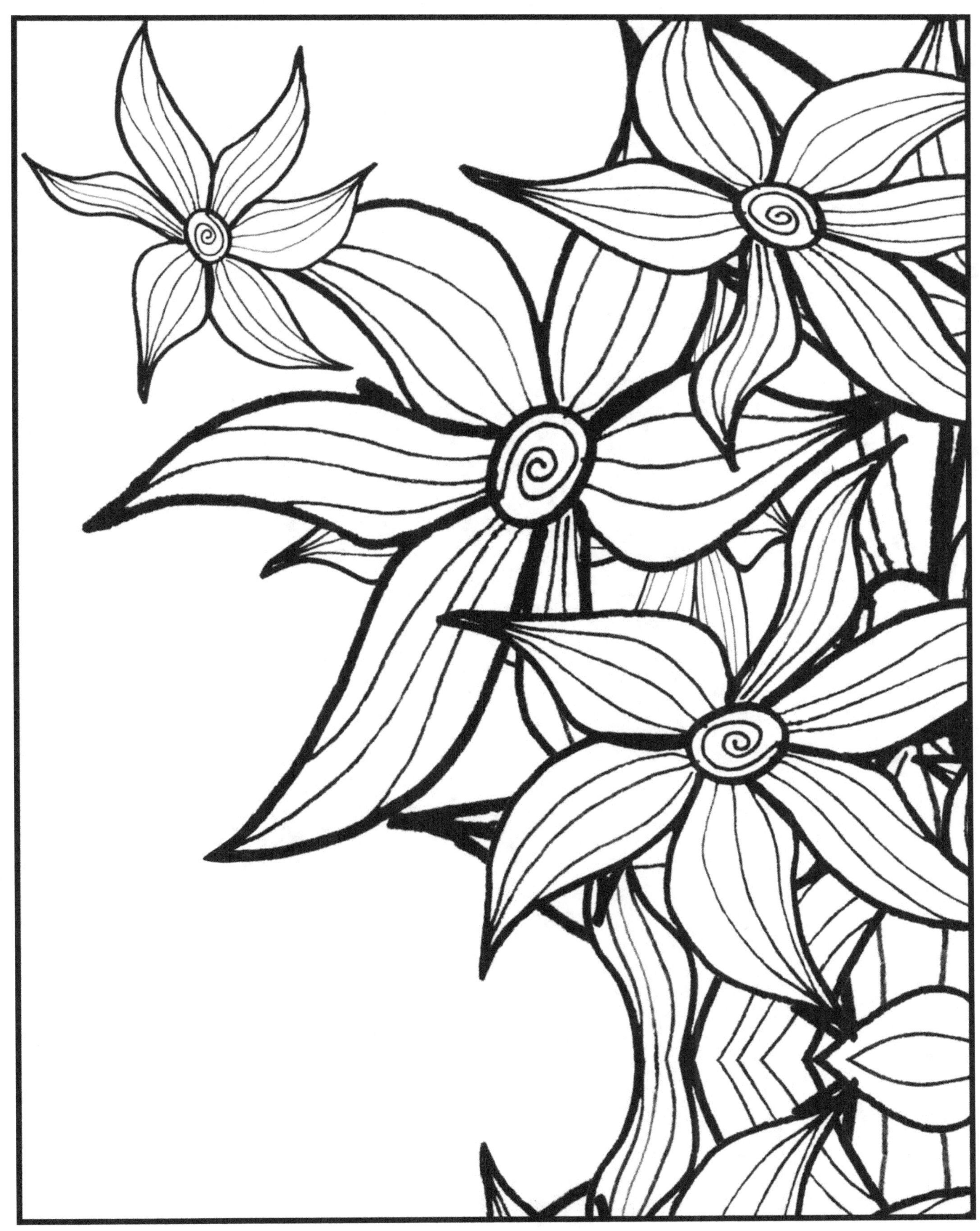

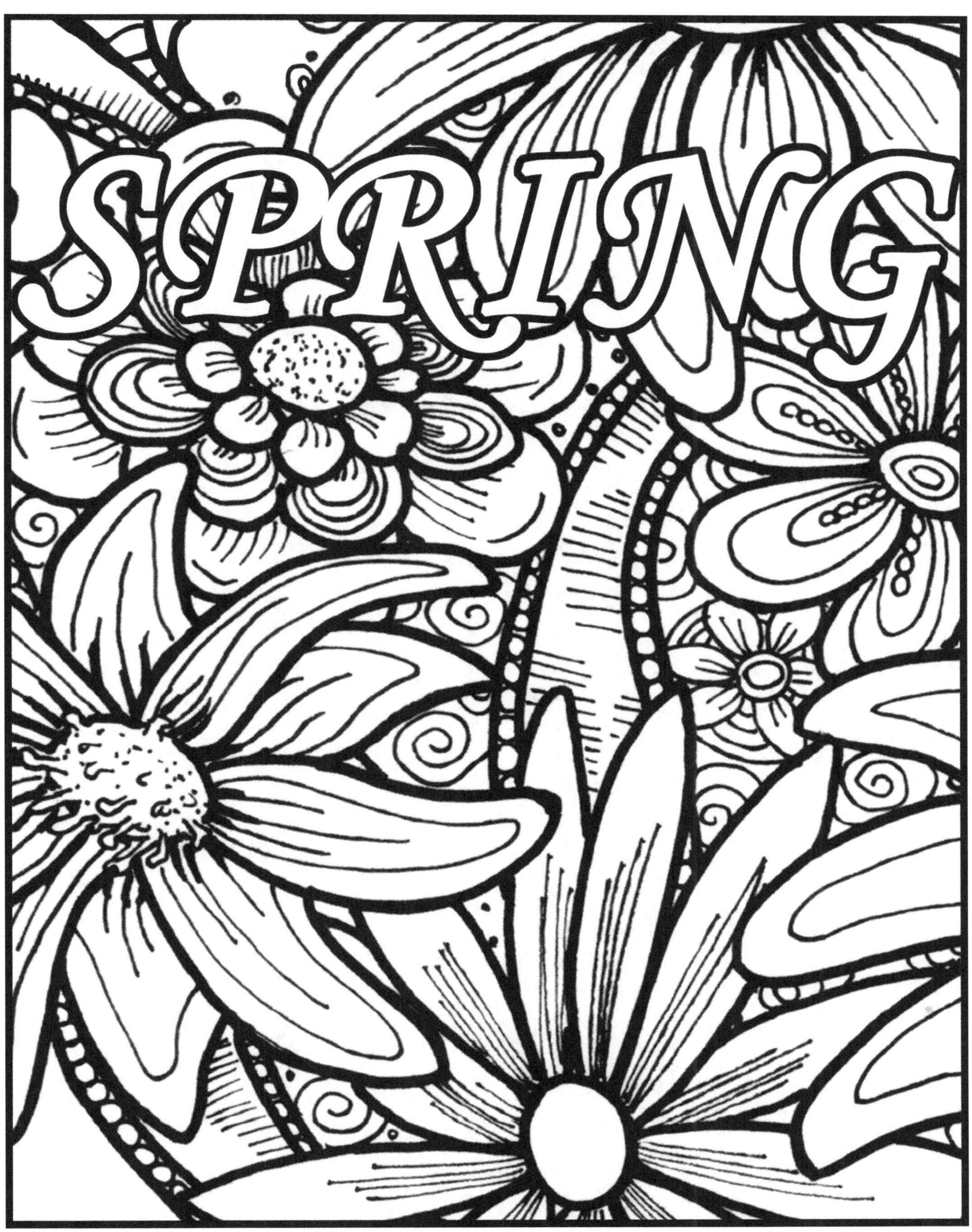
SPRING

Dear reader,
Thank you so much for purchasing my book,
I hope you enjoyed it.
I will appreciate it if you can leave a review on Amazon.

**Keep calm
and stay safe!**

Hope to see you soon.
Alex

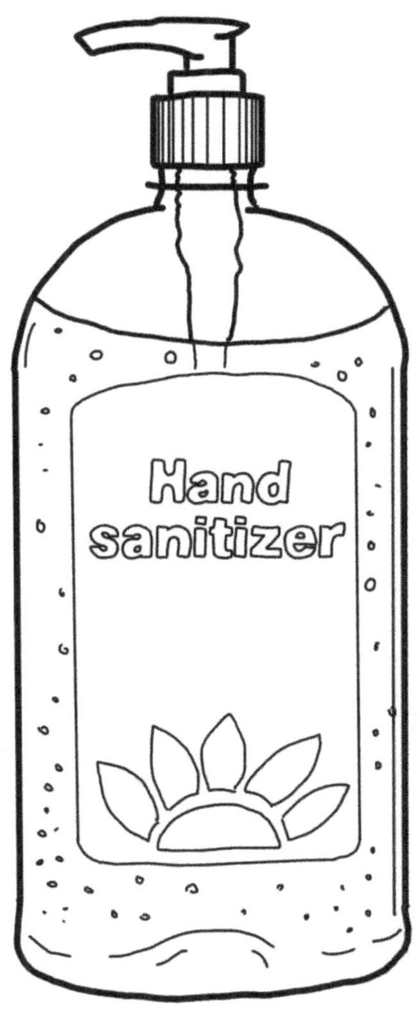


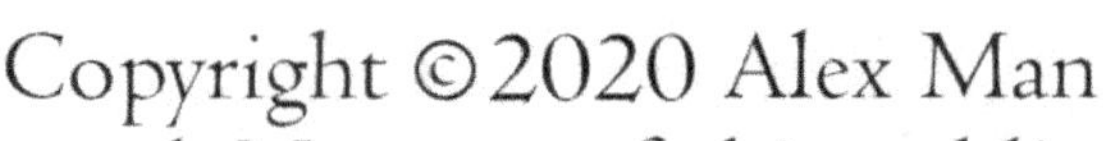